NUTRITION NUGGETS

AND MORE

BY RONDA GATES

© 1990, Ronda Gates, Lifestyles 4 Heart Press
P. O. Box 1843
Lake Oswego, OR 97035

Cover Design, Layout and Pasteup by Pat Haniford
Cartoons by Peg O'Connor
Printing by Catalogs Unlimited, Inc. Hillsboro, OR 97123
First printing November, 1989
Second printing February, 1990

ISBN 1-878319-00-0

Lifestyles by Ronda Gates® is an Oregon based corporation providing a
variety of health promotion lectures and workshops, personal growth
seminars and a weight management course to public, corporate, educational
and industrial communities.

DEDICATION

To Rebecca and Caleb, who continue to delight me...

TABLE OF CONTENTS

ACKNOWLEDGEMENTS

I always wonder who are those people that are acknowledged in books? Why is the list so long? I learned this is the way to say thanks to the people who stand by the author in the birthing of a book. I have many to acknowledge.

To the people who have supported my personal and professional growth these past ten years, especially Covert Bailey and Lea Bishop whose knowledge and mentorship stimulated my ongoing interest in nutrition...

To Caroline Derrickson and Anne Wilson-Schaef and my friends in the 12-step community who share my journey...

To John Kalbrener for his editing skills that make my writing better reading...

To Pat Haniford whose patience and long hours gave me just what I wanted...

To Peg O'Connor for putting my humor into pictures...

To Marie Livingston for recipe development...

To Anita Hoffart for analyzing the recipes...

To Jack Cornelius who always said, "I'll be right over." when the computer was contrary...

To the students, clients and audiences who continue to listen to the evolving nature of my work...

To my housemate, Sharon, who did not use her consumate acting skills on our stage during the birthing process. She remained honest and just let me be...

I give my thanks and love.

INTRODUCTION

"How do I get started? Where can I learn more about the kinds of things you've talked about today? Has anyone written a book that will reinforce the practical information we discussed in class tonight? I liked Lowfat Lifestyle® and you didn't talk about sugar or sodium or specific fats in that book. Where can I find information on those important facets of nutrition? In addition, I'd like some information on how to interpret my cholesterol reading and want to know more about omega 3 oils. Can you put me on to something that's easy to understand?

These are the kinds of questions I hear every day as I offer lectures, classes and workshops about lifestyle change. It doesn't matter whether it is at a convention, in a health club setting, a corporation or a school – Americans want the savvy to live a lifestyle of quality as well as quantity.

I first responded to these requests when I published Lowfat Lifestyle® with Valerie Parker in 1985. Nutrition Nuggets® goes beyond the information contained in Lowfat Lifestyle® and is in response to the need for a "quick read" about the nutritional aspects of lifestyle change. The first half is a collection of newsletter articles I have written. It will give you some basic information about dieting and how to choose foods wisely, including how to read labels to help you get fat and sugar out of your diet and fiber into it. You will learn about salt and cholesterol and saturated fats and dining out and stocking in and you will be introduced to some new ways to look at exercise. That information is followed by some quick-to-fix time tested recipes developed by my staff and students as more low fat cooking ingredients became available on supermarket shelves.

About half way into the book you will discover the remaining pages are upside down. That's because learning how to choose foods and beginning to live a more physically active lifestyle is only half the story. My experience is that when people make changes in the way they eat and exercise it affects other areas of their life. Changes occur. It's about new beginnings. So flip this book over to find a companion to Nutrition Nuggets® which is "the rest of the story"!

To our continued growth and good health!

ABOUT DIETS

Do you want to lose weight? If so, you are not alone. From Scarsdale to Beverly Hills, Mayo Clinic to Hilton Head, Palm Beach to New York, Americans by the millions are eating grapefruit, taking pills, adding fiber, increasing vitamins, counting calories, heightening feminism and combining foods in an ongoing, desperate effort to find a magic short cut to weight loss. Supermarket shelves groan under the weight of new products that promise good taste and fewer calories. If our responses to the problem of overfatness don't work, many of us resort to surgery in an effort to cut, staple or suck our way to success. Weight, or getting rid of it, is now a $20 billion-a-year industry that encompasses medical, emotional, entrepreneurial and spiritual issues and confronts one in every three of us.

My dictionary defines diet as a way of choosing food. So many authors have tied their name to ways of choosing foods, with emphasis on losing weight quickly, that "diet" has become a misnomer for weight loss plans. These plans emphasize weight loss, not fat loss.

Whenever I am told somone lost ten pounds in two weeks I ask, "ten pounds of what?", because it is impossible to lose more than two pounds of fat a week.

Many diets focus on low calorie levels. It is important to understand that calories aren't really "in" any food; they are a measure of the amount of energy that food can provide when it is broken down in the body. Calories can do only three things: get burned in muscle cells, keep body heat stable and all systems functioning (basal metabolic rate) or, if in excess, get stored as fat.

A pound of fat is 3,500 calories. If you burn 250 calories during exercise and eat 250 calories less a day you lose only one pound of fat a week. If that is so, how can we rely on diets that offer quicker results?

Low Calorie Diets
Most health professionals agree a woman needs a minimum of 1000-1200 calories a day and a man needs a minimum of 1500-1700 calories a day to provide the fifty or so nutrients you need daily. It is easy to calculate why diets that drop below these levels cannot provide the nutrients we need and still allow for the empty calories that are a part of all but the strictest diets. Food can be separated into two parts–the nutrient dense or nutritious part and the empty calorie or non-nutritious part. A 30% fat, 10% refined sugar diet that conforms to U. S. Dietary Goals provides 40% empty, non-nutritious calories. Thus, even a balanced and varied 1200 calorie diet would supply only 720 nutritious calories–just barely the minimum the body needs to function efficiently that day.

Any time you eat less than the minimum number of calories you need daily, your body struggles to survive the ordeal by going into a metabolic tailspin that activates lipoprotein lipase, an enzyme that encourages caloric thrift and fat hoarding. The body says, "How can I save what I'll need later in this famine?"

Diets that are often at "near starvation" levels work only temporarily. True, they are low enough in calories for some loss of body fat. They are often also low enough in carbohydrates to cause weight loss of non-fat, calorie burning muscle or other protein tissue (which breaks down to supply glucose, the body's sugar supply, to the brain).

This "making of new sugar" results in a shift of body fluids to prevent the toxicity that results from the breakdown of this non-fat tissue. Ron Deutsch, a writer famous for interpreting nutrition for the layman says, "The body consumes its own meat to get needed protein and carbohydrate." Overexercising, which usually accompanies these diets, burns more glucose than fat, and the result is the same—breakdown of protein. When this non-fat, calorie burning muscle and accompanying water weight is lost, the numbers on the scale are lower, but the total body fat percentage actually increases, leaving the dieter ounces lighter, but actually fatter. The repeated fasting and feasting these diets encourage can set up metabolic warfare that screws up metabolism so badly it is difficult to eat healthfully without gaining weight.

High Protein Diets
In 1989 low calorie, high protein diets soared in popularity when television viewers watched Oprah Winfrey lose 60 pounds on a medically monitored protein-sparing fast. Marketing geniuses were quick to capitalize on recycling the quick weight loss concept that has been around for twenty years. This diet is no different than any other quick weight loss diet. The metabolic consequences of "starving" the body of calories, whether protein is included in the diet or not, are described in the previous paragraphs. New resarch confirms there are herculean demands put on the kidney and liver system of a body struggling to survive on less than 1200 calories (for women) or 1500 (for men) and zapped with a lot of protein. The popular "formula" diets which are an outgrowth of these high protein diets, are rarely nutritionally complete, usually contain no food, and can cause constipation, gas, diarrhea, nausea and abdominal cramps. That is a

lousy way to feel, regardless of how much you want to lose weight.

Single Or Combination Food Diets

In recent years the recommendations of the best authorities on weight loss have been challenged by physicians, movie stars and self-proclaimed nutritionists from "universities" that exist only by mail. These "experts" say they have learned that bananas or grapefruit or some other secret no one has ever discovered before is the key to permanent weight loss. Dr. Frederick Stare, Professor of the Department of Nutrition at Harvard reminds us: "No one food by itself provides good nutrition." Diets that focus on one food or tell us to eat certain foods in special combinations at specific times of the day ignore this most basic principle. It takes a balanced and varied diet of two servings of food from the meat and dairy groups and four to eight servings from the bread/cereal and fruit/vegetable groups to supply the fifty or so nutrients we need every day. Diets that suggest adding vitamin or mineral tablets to supplement these miracle plans don't work because only foods can supply all the structural materials in the proper amounts needed to maintain, build and repair body tissues.

Added Fiber Diets

Dietary recommendations to add fiber to the diet in the form of powders or tablets are often the source of nutrition inaccuracies and myths that infer fiber has some magical power to eliminate appetite. Fiber is a form of indigestible starch that does make us feel full, but most people who struggle with their weight do not eat because they are hungry. They eat to satisfy an emotional hunger and to support habits that are fully integrated into a society that uses food to respond to a host of emotional needs. Fiber provides the binders and scrubbers that contribute to good gastrointestinal health. But the best source for this calorie free part of food is in its original state, attached to food rather than as bulk powders added to foods or tablets taken before meals.

The reason added fiber diets don't work is because most people don't eat because they are hungry. Feeling full contributes little to whether or not a person who struggles with weight chooses to put food in his or her mouth.

Packaged Food Diets
For the dieter who wants some structure while learning new ways to pick and choose from the four food groups, there are diets provided as packaged foods which are designed to provide that structure–along with high profits for the manufacturer and distributor of the food product. Packaged diet foods can get you started but do not teach the new patterns that encourage lifetime habits. In fact they begin a pattern of dependency on the packaged product and system. The serving size of these convenient-to-prepare foods are usually quite small. These small portions ignore the emotional and psychological needs and compulsions that influence overeating, and they treat only the symptoms of overfatness. They do nothing to contribute to changing the lifestyle that leads to and maintains overfatness.

Single Focus Diets
Diseases of overfatness fill our hospitals yet some diets continue to focus on eliminating only salt or food additives or cholesterol or suggest using one fat or oil over another. These diets are ignoring what respected health professionals describe as the most dangerous additive in our diet today–fat. Fat is fat. Decreasing total fat in the diet from current levels of about 45% to recommended levels of 30% is the goal. (The goal itself is not about whether the fat is saturated, polyunsaturated or monounsaturated, although there are recommendations to keep saturated fats to 10% of total fat intake.) There is a study that shows that over a four month period of time a 20% fat, 1200 calorie diet generates more fat loss than a 45% fat, 1200 calorie diet. That sets calorie counters back on their ears. Lowering *total* fat intake is the answer to achieving optimum health and reasonable weight goals.

Long term success on any weight loss plan requires a change in attitude coupled with education, preferably as one of a group of people who provide one another with the underlying support needed to integrate and change from the old you to the new you. The diet you create must be one you can live with and thrive on–for the rest of your life.

When you evaluate a diet, ask yourself: is the product/ book/person promising something that seems too good to be true? Do I have to buy a product or book that promises this method and/or product alone can cure overweight? Does the diet rely on testimonials and case histories rather than scientific data to support claims? Has it been reviewed by qualified experts with recognized nutrition degrees from reputable universities?

Fit Or Fat author, Covert Bailey, adds advice that has been adopted by all reputable diet counselors: "Without exercise even the most balanced diet is attacking only half the problem. Eating smaller quantities while maintaining a balanced and varied diet, combined with aerobic exercise, is the only safe and effective way to lose fat weight. You have to change your body *metabolism,* how your body uses calories."

The story of the tortoise and the hare is a useful metaphor to demonstrate how to eat to take fat off and keep it off. Although success is more tortoise than hare-like, it is success, the kind of permanent success that comes from daily persistence and small changes over a long period of time. The goal, after all, is to lose fat, not our mind! Dr. Jean Mayer, president of Tufts University, offers the most consistent and upbeat overview: "A good diet is not only one which will contribute to your health but also one which should help you maintain you in good cheer."

Bon Appetit!

ON RATING
DIETS

It is virtually impossible to lose more than two pounds of body *fat* per week. Any diet that promises pound loss of more than that is eventually going to crash. Despite this, the $20 billion weight loss industry continues to try to get you to part with your dieting dollars. With very few exceptions, their diet plans are all crash diets.

Losing fat permanently means more than buying formulas and products that trick your body into achieving a scale weight that makes you smile. It requires more than simply choosing and/or combining foods in "magic" ways, or eating specific items at certain times of the day. *Permanent* weight loss means understanding that your body functions optimally when it is exercised regularly and fed sensibly, following the U.S. Dietary Goals that have been around so long that most of us take them for granted. These goals include: eating less fat, cholesterol, sugar and salt, and choosing food with more fiber and complex carbohydrates. That means eating more fruits and vegetables and whole grains, as well as choosing meats, poultry, fish and dairy products that are low in fat.

The personal key to permanent weight loss is finding your personal combination of diet, exercise and lifestyle changes that you can implement and sustain *for your lifetime*. It is learning about the physiological and psychological issues that have prevented success in the past, and noticing which of your behaviors are self-supporting and which are self de-feating, so you can reinforce your self-support and stop defeating yourself.

Each time I meet with a new group of "dieters" who register for my weight management class, most of them confess to a long history of dieting. They admit they are there because they have learned there are no short cuts to losing weight and that "diets don't work". They sense there is something more. Most enter class saying, "I know what I need to do; I just can't do it." Some have gone to reputable professionals and have learned about nutrition as well as how to choose foods. Each dieter has experienced some degree of success–inevitably followed by a return to old patterns, including their old weight gain patterns. These unhappy and disappointed di-eters empathise with one another as each tells his or her story of multiple attempts to lose weight on a variety of diet and exercise programs. Eventually they all agree they didn't work because they were on "crash" diets, designed for short term goals–and they did not address self-defeating behav-iors.

For many years people whose eating habits were "out of control" came to me for help. They talked about their lack of will power and the need to get their lives "under control". They wanted me to share my technique for management of their weight. I prescribed diets and designed their exercise programs every step of the way. It gave them an illusion of their own control and it worked–for awhile. When they returned to me months later for more help, or to get another "fix", or to be remotivated, I had to look at what went wrong. Many factors contributed to their long term lack of success. But underlying all the emotional and psychological issues around choosing foods I came to a new understanding of why almost all diets–including those I recommended–do not work in the long run. What I learned was that the techniques I was using were *mine* – not *theirs*; the techniques I prescribed were integrated into *my* particular being, but did not fit *their* particular beings. Eventually they returned to their own self-defeating habits.

I believe the key to permanent lifestyle change (including weight management) is knowing yourself well enough to be able to develop your *own* technique for "dieting", rather than following the rules someone else may give you. My job now is to assist people in recognizing that I cannot give them an "answer." I can guide them through a process of self-evaluation and self-discovery that will allow them to know and claim themselves. For some, that is a lengthy process filled with much noticing and awareness of personal patterns combined with a commitment (*not* will power) to make and sustain change in the face of a family and a society that may like the status quo. When these "diet junkies" come to me looking for an answer, one of my tasks is to help them become aware of why, physiologically and psychologically, *there are no quick answers*. In this process I teach them practical tools for choosing a diet in keeping with dietary goals, focusing on decreasing sugar and fat and increasing fiber.

They learn about balance and variety in a diet and how to assure sufficient calories. We explore the ways an exercise program suited to their bodies and schedules can fulfill their wants and needs for self-care. We also spend a lot of time exploring behavior patterns, because noticing how we operate in the world is essential in the process of making change. We explore family of origin issues, practice assertiveness, clarify values, structure our support system and affirm our new habits. In time the changes they choose to make in the way they choose foods and dietary habits, combined with changes in how they operate in the world, add up to successes, achievement of short term goals and the ongoing motivation to continue. With support they make more and more choices that elevate their self-esteem. And when they "fall off the wagon" they are encouraged to honor where they are and avoid one of their oldest long term patterns, the pattern of judging themselves.

There are times when I provide a "diet" for clients. When I do it is to help them find the time to develop the coping skills necessary for determining and making their own changes. And I do it with their input at every step.

One of the tools that is useful to my students is learning how to rate a diet. We ask the following questions; they will help you scrutinize diet plans and choose one that can help you lose fat and not your mind.

Ronda's Diet Rating Checklist.

_____1. Does the diet promise quick weight loss results?
Crash diets promise quick payoffs but don't mention the long-term penalty of weight re-gain and the inability to eat as many calories as you did before the diet started. Instead, set a realistic and healthy goal of a gradual weight loss of one or two pounds per week.

_____2. Does the diet depend on one food or product to work?
A healthy, well-balanced diet includes a _variety_ of foods from the four food groups to supply you with the 50 or so nutrients you need every day.

_____3. Does the diet have sufficient calories to provide the nutrients you need daily?
While dieting, women need to eat at least 1,000 to 1,200 low in fat calories per day; men 1,500 to 1,700. Starvation-level diets (approximately 600 calories for women and 800 for men) work only temporarily because the body attempts to save what it can during what it perceives as a "famine."

_____4. Does the diet demand you eat certain foods at certain times of the day?
This kind of diet ignores your lifestyle and food preferences and may prove too difficult or inconvenient to follow. Do not look for a "diet"–think lifestyle change.

_____5. Who promotes or endorses the diet?
Look for endorsement by reputable dietitians or nutritionists; pass up diets promoted by paid media personalities (actors!) or individuals with degrees from dubious institutions.

_____6. Does the author or ad claim to have found the diet secret that no one else has ever discovered?
If so, the diet is either ignoring or is ignorant of the great amount of solid, verified and re-verified scientific research about weight loss. Instead, trust yourself and, keep looking; choose a diet well grounded in nutritional fact and scientific data.

_____7. Are behavior issues addressed in the plan?
Although learning to choose foods more healthily is helpful to most people, food is rarely the issue for those of us who struggle with our weight on a daily basis. That is why weight loss is rarely permanent. External cues play a powerful role in our decisions to eat or not-to-eat and the foods we choose to satisfy our physical and emotional hunger. Addressing behavior issues with pretty place settings or eating in a proper environment or keeping food out of sight are valid beginning tools for supporting lifestyle change. However, long term weight management has more to do with choices we make when faced with the daily events that trigger the use or misuse of food in the first place. It's about the family systems and patterns of coping that may keep us comfortable, but not mentally or physically healthy. Learning to notice those daily events that

trigger the use of food, instead of feelings, to re-solve issues is a first step. From there behavior change requires a lengthy and patient process of small changes. With the support of people who care about you that is not only possible but sat-isfying and transforming.

Regardless of your next course of action, remember: dieting has to do with how you choose foods, not how much you weigh. It's not only the bites of foods, it's the bites of life. In the chapters that follow may you find the morsels, meals and mindfulness that bring you personal pleasure – for the rest of your life.

OVER FAT OR OVERWEIGHT?

"You want me to do *what*?", Ruth asked, looking aghast. "How will I know if I am losing weight?"

I had just suggested the members of my weight management class throw away their scales in favor of having their body fat measured.

"Tell me you're kidding," Donna pleaded. "I don't want to know how much fat I have on my body. Ugh!"

I was not surprised at the reaction of the class to the possibility of learning their percent of body fat. Fat is a loaded issue for our society. We have been lead to believe it is bad to have fat on our bodies, and too much of our life energy has been spent on quick ways to get rid of it. My experience is that very few people have any concept of how much fat or non-fat they carry on their bodies.

"How many of you weigh yourselves every day?" I asked. Every hand went up. I knew the routine. I had done it myself too many times. Up in the morning, stumble to the bathroom, empty the bladder, off with the night clothes, then step on the scale. I would look down and take the first reading of the day. No matter where the needle fell I stepped off the scale, adjusted it precisely to zero, stepped on it again and did my first dance of the day—hoping to nudge the needle lower. If the scale registered a lower number than I hoped for, I broke into my first smile of the day. I knew I could eat whatever I wanted. If the number was higher than I hoped, a mild depression would overtake me. Some of the time I would berate myself for something I may have enjoyed eating the previous day. I thought of myself as "fat" and went through the day depriving myself of what I really wanted (because I didn't deserve it) and eating what I now describe as "rabbit food"—lettuce and carrot sticks and low fat cottage cheese.

I told my class that I was one of the growing number of health promotion specialists who are encouraging others to throw away their scales. That is because a scale will not tell you how fat you are. It will tell you how much you weigh but the number on the scale is not an indication of how much of your weight is fat. Weight is no longer the issue in determining optimum health; whether you are or are not at risk to a number of fat-related diseases depends on the amount and ratio of fat on your body. Instead of using height-weight charts to determine realistic weight goals these professionals are evaluating our muscle-to-fat ratio and recommending goals of 20-25% on women's bodies and 15-20% on men's bodies. When I told the class that the average person I "test" is about ten points over those goals they were not eager to see where they fell on my statistical scale.

I asked them to trust me. "Knowing your body fat percentage can be a valuable piece of information to people who want to lose fat weight," I explained. It's not only a basis for measuring changes, we can also use the "numbers" to determine realistic weight goals. Here's how:

Suppose you are a male who weighs 200 pounds. When I

measure your body fat it is 22%. To calculate your pounds of
fat we will multiply your current weight by your percent of
body fat.

200 (current weight) x .22 (percent of body fat)
= 44 (pounds of fat)

To calculate your pounds of non-fat or lean mass, subtract
your pounds of fat from you current weight.

200 (current weight) – 44 (pounds of fat)
= 156 (pounds of non-fat or lean mass).

You are approximately 156 pounds of lean, 44 pounds of fat.
When you lose weight you do not want to lose lean mass. You
already learned that your lean mass includes the valuable
muscle that burns the calories your body uses for energy.
Instead you want to retain your current lean mass and decrease body fat from its current level of 22% to a goal of 15%.
At that point your current lean mass will be 85% of your body
weight.

100% total body weight – 15% fat weight = 85% lean mass

To determine your realistic weight goal, divide the current
lean weight (156) by .85 (the percentage of your desired body
lean mass goal).

$$\frac{156}{.85} = 183.5 \text{ pounds}$$

The resulting number, 183.5, is a realistic weight goal. You
can determine how much fat you have to lose by subtracting
your realistic weight goal from your current weight.

200 (current weight) – 183.5 (realistic weight)
= 16.5 pounds of fat to lose

Here is another example. This time suppose a woman whose
current body weight is 150 pounds has a desired body fat

goal of 25%. When she has her body fat measured she learns she is 30% fat. To calculate her pounds of fat multiply her current weight by her percent of body fat.

150 (current weight) x .30 (percent of body fat)
= 45 (pounds of fat)

To calculate her pounds of non-fat or lean mass subtract her pounds of fat from her current weight.

150 (current weight) − 45 (pounds of fat)
= 105 (pounds of non-fat or lean mass)

When this woman decreases her body fat from 30% to 25% her lean mass will comprise 75% of her body weight.

100% total body weight − 25% fat weight = 75% lean mass.

To determine a realistic weight goal for this individual divide the current lean (105) by .75 (the percentage of her desired lean mass goal).

$$\frac{105}{.75} = 140 \text{ pounds}$$

The resulting number, 140, is a realistic weight goal. She can determine how much fat she has to lose by subtracting her realistic weight goal from her current weight.

150 (current weight) − 140 (realistic weight)
= 10 pounds of fat to lose

"Isn't that neat?" I asked the class. "Isn't that a lot better than looking at height-weight charts that don't take into account the amount of lean, calorie burning muscle on your body?" They agreed it was–especially when I told them that most people who carry excess pounds have a higher than average lean mass and reminded them that it's lean mass that burns calories.

They lined up.

In <u>Lowfat Lifestyle</u>* I encouraged readers to get their body fat measured and I described two methods for doing so. Since then other methods are on the scene. It seems appropriate to update my information.

Hydrostatic Weighing continues to be the gold standard for the measurement of body fat; all other methods are not considered useful unless they correlate closely with hydrostatic results. Although hydrostatic weighing can be the most accurate way to measure your body's fat/lean composition there are some disadvantages to this method. It involves exhaling fully (because air weighs as fat in this procedure) while you are completely submerged in a tank of water. At the same time you must hold still until an experienced technician can get a reading on an overhead scale. This is a somewhat uncomfortable procedure for some people, especially if they are asthmatic or afraid of being submerged in water. Since the density of your body is proportional to the amount of body fat, a sophisticated equation converts the scale reading to numbers that can tell you how much fat and lean tissue you have. If you have a skilled and experienced technician who will encourage and help you at the same time s/he takes an accurate reading from a scale that is often less than still—you will get the most accurate measurement of your lean-to-fat ratio. Under these circumstances hydrostatic weighing can be a powerful motivator for making the necessary exercise and diet changes to reach optimum body fat goals.

The **Skinfold** or "pinch" test is the most common way body fat is measured. A skinfold caliper pinches and measures the amount of subcutaneous fat on several parts of the body. Using a sophisticated formula these measurements are converted to body density and subsequently to percent of body fat. The sites used in the pinch are dependent upon the

* See page 16 of <u>LOWFAT LIFESTYLE</u>.

protocol used, but the most common sites include the bicep or front of the upper arm, tricep or back of the upper arm, sub-scapular which means under the shoulder blade, iliac crest which is where the hip bone is most prominent near the waist and/or thigh and pectoral or upper chest region. Most errors in this method occur because the technician varies the pressure of the pinch by the caliper from site to site or when repeating the measurement. There is now an electronic skin-fold caliper which helps remove technical errors from this test and makes it relatively accurate and simple to perform in many settings.

Electrical Impedence is the most popular of the newest methods for measuring body fat. It is fast, convenient and fairly accurate if you haven't hydrated or dehydrated your body lately. Impedence is the measurement of any resistance in the flow of an electrical current passed between an electrode on your right hand and another on your right foot. This procedure is based on the principle that water conducts electrical current. Assuming the body's muscle tissues contain approximately 70% water, the electrical current will use the muscle tissues as a path for the current, instead of passing through the fat which contains very little water. When the current flows freely there is no resistance. Any impedence to the flow of the current is measured and related to your total body weight. The disadvantage to this method is that the results are not always repeatable because fluid shifts in the body so rapidly. The advantage is that it is quick and non-invasive.

Ultrasound is another quick and non-invasive method of body fat testing that is popular because it is easy to use at any location. A very mild sound wave is passed through your body at the mid-thigh and the waist. This sophisticated instrument measures the density of body fat at those points. Then, using a complex mathematical formula, it calculates percent of body fat and other interesting (but relatively useless information) on a lengthy computer printout. As with the impedence method, results aren't always repeatable.

Regardless of what method you use, don't focus on the numbers. If you are tested using more than one method don't make yourself crazy comparing the varying results. Chose one of them and use that result to set a goal, then try to get the same technician to repeat the same measurements under similar conditions after you have embarked on your lifestyle changes for a few months. If you have stuck to your lower-in-fat diet and aerobic exercise program you will see dramatic proof that the inches you have lost have also contributed to your health.

ABOUT FAT CELLS

1. Everyone is born with a certain number of fat cells.
   (Some are born with more than others.)
2. Fat cells are permanent.
   (Although some fat cells can be removed by liposuction.)
3. More fat cells, which also will not disappear, can be
   formed:

   in the first weeks of life
   in periods of rapid growth (adolescence)
   during pregnancy
   in periods of excessive or rapid weight gain.
4. Fat cells are determined to be as full as possible.
5. The only way to empty your fat cells is with regular
   moderate aerobic exercise and a low fat diet.
   (Overexercising or a too low in calorie diet stimulates
   the fat cells to grab on to any incoming calories or retain
   whatever fat is already stored there.)

ABOUT LEAN MASS

To maintain or increase body lean mass (muscle) you must:
1. exercise aerobically
2. lift weights
3. eat sufficient calories.

QUICK STARTS

Have you made a commitment to a lifestyle change? If so, one of the obstacles you face may be a level of enthusiasm that can sustain change for the short, but not the long term. I prefer not to tell others what to eat but I am willing to be a guide and coach on the quest for knowledge that assures the changes are personal and can be integrated into individual lifestyles. Each time I give a lecture one of my primary goals is to help my audience recognize how a diet too high in fat, sugar, and alcohol hampers their quest for optimum physical (and mental) health. I encourage them to avoid foods that are at least 80% fat and I provide them with a list of some of these high in fat, empty calorie foods. "Begin noticing how often these foods show up in your daily diet," I suggest. "Look for lower in fat substitutes that will satisfy you. They are available." My list is on the following page. If these foods are a part of your diet you, too, have an opportunity to "grow leaner".

Butter, 100% fat	Avocado, 90% fat
Margarine, 100% fat	Half and Half Cream, 80% fat
Vegetable oil, 100% fat	Sour Cream, 85% fat
Mayonnaise, 99% fat	Cheddar Cheese, 84% fat
Whipped Cream, 96% fat	Brick Cheese, 80% fat
Olives, 95% fat	Hollandaise Sauce, 78% fat
Cream Cheese, 90% fat	Most Nuts, 80% fat

Here are some substitutes for the foods listed above as well as other quick start tips and reminders to help you begin to change the way you eat:

Avoid gravies, fatty sauces and creamed foods.

Ninety percent of the calories in most salad dressings are fat. Use reduced calorie mayonnaise and sour cream, low fat and non-fat yogurt or lowfat buttermilk to make dressings from scratch or to dilute purchased salad dressings.

Add at least one piece of fruit to your daily food intake.

Begin thinking of high fat foods such as whole milk cheese as a treat. When you want cheese, use the part skim or other low fat varieties.

Avoid processed meats. They are high in fat (and salt).

Invest in non-stick surfaced pans or before cooking, spray your pans with a non-stick vegetable spray. You won't have to use so much grease to prepare your foods.

Enjoy the natural flavor of vegetables with a sprinkling of herbs or a squeeze of lemon juice instead of margarine, butter or other high fat sauces. Purchase and use one of the sprinkle-on butter alternatives like Molly McButter for hot foods.

Purchase a variety of spices and herbs (like Mrs. Dash products) available in the seasoning section of your supermarket and use them to flavor your recipes.

Trim excess fat off meat and remove the skin and underlying fat from any chicken dishes you prepare.

When you prepare meals begin thinking of meat as a condiment rather than the main dish. Stretch your meal with pasta, beans, rice or other grains. You will soon enjoy letting starches and vegetables take center stage.

Cut the fat in your favorite recipes from a third to a half. Look for new recipes that use much less fat.

Cut **back** (I didn't say cut out!) sugar, honey, molasses, jams, jellies, candy, ice cream and soft drinks. These foods are high in empty calories and so lacking in nutrients that, like the high fat foods listed above, they do not deserve to be called a food.

Be aware that vegetarianism can be an unhealthy way to eat if it includes a lot of high fat foods or if it is too low in calories. If you choose to eat this way, be sure you know how to get all the nutrients your body needs to function healthily for a *long* time.

Don't skip any meals. Deprivation as a way of losing weight does not work.

Notice when you are hungry and satisfy that hunger. And, notice when you are full and quit eating.

Get in the leftover habit. You *don't* have to finish everything on your plate—or everything you cook. One of my favorite breakfasts is leftovers from dinner the night before.

Alcohol is called an empty calorie food because it has no nutrients. Alcohol is also a trigger to compulsive overeating for many people and can be a powerful barrier to maintaining a commitment to healthy eating. If you enjoy an occasional glass of wine, champagne, sherry or a beer, be sure to plan your day to allow for these empty calories, and be aware of the role it plays in your choice of foods. If you drink more than one glass, alternate it with a glass of mineral water or another non-alcoholic beverage.

Exercise is crucial to weight loss and maintaining weight loss. If you have never exercised before start walking! More and more diseases of longevity are being traced to a lifestyle of poor diet and lack of exercise that may have its origins early in life. Thomas Jefferson said it best: "Walking is the best exercise. Habituate yourself to walk very far."

If you do nothing more than follow these guidelines you will notice a significant change in the way you feel in a few days and the way you look and feel in a couple of months.

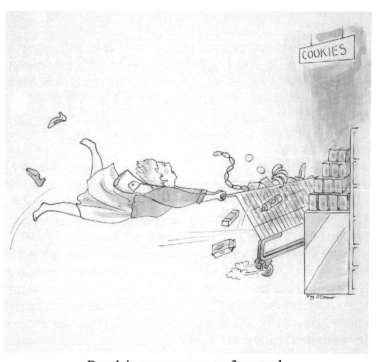

Ronda's cart went out of control
when it got to the dessert aisle.

FATTY BLOOD

Jerry checked in at the first session of a Lifestyles weight management class with a goal to drop twenty pounds and lower his cholesterol level. He told me that several months ago his wife dragged him into the local supermarket and turned him over to a white-coated technician who, for a fee of $7, pricked his finger, sent a drop of his blood through a machine and, in less than five minutes presented him with an elevated total cholesterol level of 230. Since that test much of Jerry's waking and all his eating time had been focused on worrying about "lowering his cholesterol". After six weeks on a "low cholesterol" diet, his repeat test showed a level of 224. He was frustrated. When I asked him if he knew what the number meant he admitted didn't–he just knew it was high and cholesterol was "bad". Jerry's partly right.

Cholesterol is a fatty molecule that is essential to life. Like the beams that support the walls in your home, it gives structure to the walls of your cells and plays an important role in hormonal functions and digestion. Cholesterol only becomes villainous in excessive amounts when it accelerates the accumulation of fatty plaque on artery walls, hardening and narrowing them. Medically it is called atherosclerosis. When the plaque pinches the channel shut, blood, with its vital supply of oxygen and nutrients, can no longer swish through. When that happens in an artery leading to the heart, it results in a heart attack. When it happens in an artery leading to the brain, it results in a stroke.

Because it is a fat, cholesterol isn't soluble in water or blood. Like all fat, it floats. To make it soluble in blood, this fat, with the scientific description "lipo", is coated or surrounded by protein. It is then called a lipo-protein. The more protein that coats a glob of cholesterol, the greater its density. Cholesterol with a thicker or more dense coating of protein is called High Density Lipoprotein cholesterol or HDL cholesterol and is less inclined to stick to artery walls. Studies indicate it also has a scavenger effect on plaque; it hauls other cholesterol out of cell walls then takes it to the liver where it is excreted in the bile or used in digestion or in making hormones. Cholesterol with little protein is called Low Density Lipoprotein cholesterol or LDL cholesterol and tends to be sticky–and it adheres to artery walls leading to the atherosclerosis I described above.

The finger stick procedure Larry experienced is a screening method that is useful for the initial evaluation of total blood cholesterol levels. It is a much needed effort to identify people with this problem. Desirable total cholesterol blood levels are less than 200 (milligrams per deciliter). If the reading is 200-239 it is described as borderline high. Anytime a cholesterol level is elevated above 240 it is considered high and the risk of coronary heart disease is almost double than that at a reading of 200.

The accuracy of a finger stick (as opposed to a more comprehensive lipid [fat] profile done after a 12 hour fast) is subject to a significant error. If you receive a report that indicates a high level you will be encouraged to repeat the test at a later date under the care of a physician. This is when you will want to ask your doctor for a lipid profile which breaks out the types of cholesterol into the HDL and LDL levels. If your cholesterol total is high because of a lot of HDL that is no problem, because high HDL levels are known to lower the risk of heart disease. Recommended levels of HDL cholesterol are 45 and higher for men, 55 and higher for women. However, if your total cholesterol is high because of elevated levels of LDL it is time for lifestyle changes. Recommended levels for LDL are 100 or less. If your reading is 100-130 you are considered a borderline risk and if 130-160 at high risk for cardiac disease.

Some physicians are more interested in reporting your total cholesterol to high-density lipoprotein ratio. They recommend a ratio of 4.5 or less for men and 4 or less for women. For example: a woman having a total choesterol of 200 milligrams per 100 milliliters of blood and an HDL of 50 milligrams (200/50) would have a ratio of 4. Some physicians also look for a reading where there are three or more times HDL cholesterol than LDL cholesterol. With either of these methods if the ratio falls within normal limits the reading is satisfactory no matter what the total cholesterol measures.

Although there are medications available to lower blood cholesterol levels, the gram doses of the vitamin, niacin, recommended by many professionals and non-professionals for this use have a number of potential serious side effects and should be used only under the care of a physician who is experienced in cholesterol management. Instead I concur with experts who encourage physicians to prescribe a two faceted approach of aerobic exercise (to raise HDL levels) and a low fat diet (to decrease LDL levels) for their patients with elevated cholesterol levels.

Jerry had taken the dietary approach to treat his cholesterol and it hadn't worked. When we later reviewed his diet it became clear why. He had only been given part of the story. Like many people who try to modify a diet to lower blood lipid levels, Jerry had focused on lowering dietary cholesterol, not dietary fat. He had done so by moving from butter to margarine as a spread and by using polyunsaturated oils in his cooking instead of animal and other saturated fats.

An analysis of Jerry's diet showed that it was 41% fat–typical of the average American. He had switched from one fat to another, ignoring the little publicized fact that a high fat-low cholesterol diet is just as dangerous as a high fat-high cholesterol diet. He was stunned. Now he was eager to learn how to read food labels, modify recipes and order more prudently in restaurants. And, once he learned that aerobic exercise would improve his body's ability to breakdown fat in the blood and raise HDL cholesterol levels, he was eager to find an exercise program motivating enough to become a permanent part of his lifestyle.

Sheepishly Jerry admitted that he couldn't resist asking me about using the vitamin, niacin, or fish oil capsules he'd heard could contribute to lowering his cholesterol level. The local health food store was promoting the use of these non-prescription drugs and he wondered if I would suggest a suitable dosage for him. I couldn't.

Jerry was a diligent student and after three months he had lost ten pounds of fat, was regenerating the muscle bulk of his younger years and, best of all, his cholesterol level was 198. He also became an advocate of cholesterol testing in his business office and was enjoying his new role as a proponent of a lowfat lifestyle. As for me, I had the pleasure of watching another less than healthy individual turn his life around.

GET THE FAT OUT!

Former Surgeon General C. Everett Koop made headline news in 1989 when he announced that fat was the underlying cause of the killer diseases in our country. He reinforced U. S. Dietary Goals, as well as guidelines written by the American Dietitic Association, the American Heart Association and the American Cancer Society when he recommended we lower the fat in our diet from 45% (the equivalent of one stick of butter a day!) to 30%. And he left most of our population wondering, once again, how to do it.

If you are like most people I meet, the issues around fat create more confusion than clarity. Here is how I describe fat and why certain kinds of fats are discouraged and others are encouraged in our diet.

Fat is made up of triglycerides which can be measured in the blood to determine if a diet is too high in fat. Triglycerides get their name because they are composed of a molecule of glycerin and three (tri) molecules of fatty acids. These fatty acids are saturated, monounsaturated or polyunsaturated, depending on the number of "double" bonds in the molecule. A <u>mono</u>unsaturated fatty acid has <u>one</u> double bond and can accept hydrogen at two sites. A <u>poly</u>unsaturaated fatty acid has <u>two or more</u> double bonds and can accept multiple hydrogen at these sites.

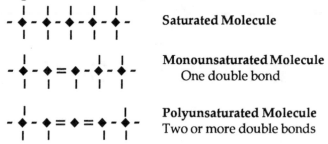

Saturated Molecule

Monounsaturated Molecule
One double bond

Polyunsaturated Molecule
Two or more double bonds

Although fat itself is generally classified as either saturated, polyunsaturated or monounsaturated, it is actually a combination of all three fatty acids in varying amounts.

Research studies show that dietary saturated fat is a primary factor in keeping blood cholesterol levels high. It is found primarily in animal products (which also contain cholesterol) and in the plant oils, palm oil and coconut oil. So Americans are encouraged to keep their intake of these fats and oils down to a minimum of 10% (1/3 of the total recommended fat of 30%).

The more saturated a fat is, the harder it is at room temperature. Hard fats holds foods together better than soft fats and the harder a fat is, the less likely it is to become rancid, making hydrogenated fat useful as an extender of shelf life of packaged foods. That is why manufacturers force hydrogen into primarily unsaturated vegetable oils. These partially hydrogenated oils are now more saturated and have a longer shelf life.

Hydrogenated, palm kernel and coconut oil, the *most* saturated and *least desirable* oils are also less expensive than other saturated fats. That is why we see so much of it on food labels.

In response to consumer advocacy many food companies are taking these highly saturated tropical oils out of their products and replacing them with partially hydrogenated soybean, cottonseed and other plant oils. This is a healthy move toward decreasing the saturated fat in our diet.

U.S. Agriculture Department lists show the saturation levels of oil. When you prepare foods you want to pick the oils with the lowest levels of saturated fats. Here are some of the more common fats and oils on the market today showing the percent of saturated fat in each. Remember, all these are 100% fat. This chart* shows only the amount of saturated and polyunsaturated fat (the remaining percentages are monounsaturated fats.)

FAT	% Saturated	% Polyunsaturated
Canola (rapeseed)	7	33
Safflower	9	75
Walnut	9	63
Sunflower	10	66
Corn	13	59
Olive	14	8
Soybean	14	58
Sesame Seed	14	42
Peanut	17	58
Soft Margarine	17	50
Hard Margarine	22	25
Cotton seed	26	52
Crisco (in can)	27	not available
Chicken Fat-Schmaltz	30	21
Pork Fat (Lard)	40	11
Palm	49	9
Beef Fat/Tallow	50	4
Butter	62	4
Cocoa Butter	60	3
Palm Kernel	81	2
Coconut	87	2

*Information from U.S. Dept. of Agriculture Bulletin No. 70

Since there are no legal restrictions on the kind of fats or oils that can be used in food products, you have to be vigilant about labeling even when you are armed with the information on the forgoing chart. Most advertising for polyunsaturated fat attempts to make an oil with higher levels of saturated fat look like a better choice. For example, corn oil is 59% polyunsaturated, whereas canola oil is only 33% polyunsaturated. With clever marketing, that could make corn oil look like a smarter buy. However, if you return to the chart on page 31 you will see that corn oil has 13% saturated fat and canola oil is only 7% saturated fat. The lower in saturated fat canola oil is a better choice.

Beware of purchasing products whose labels say "cholesterol free" or "no animal fat." On closer examination you may discover these foods contain palm, coconut or other hydrogenated oils that are cholesterol-free but high in saturated fat. Companies who label products as though your health is in their best interest are often, in fact, preparing the foods with much more concern for their profit.

Once again, the typical American diet is too high in **total** fat and contains much more cholesterol level raising saturated fat than cholesterol level lowering unsaturated fat. These are the foods high in saturated fat that you should avoid: ground beef, deep fried foods, whole milk beverages and dairy products, hot dogs, bacon, lunch meats, eggs, butter, doughnuts, cakes, cookies, ice cream and chocolate, creamy sauces and many packaged baked goods and cereals.

By decreasing your total fat intake to thirty percent, then changing the type of fat you are eating to de-emphasize saturated fats, you can join those of us who *live* the LOWFAT LIFESTYLE!

ABOUT OMEGA 3 OILS

It's in the media! We can eat salmon.

Or can we?

Researchers first became interested in "fattier" fish a few years ago when they discovered that Greenland Eskimos (who eat 3/4 pound of fish a day) and Japanese fishermen (who eat more than a quarter pound a day) have a very low rate of heart disease. (The average American eats only 13 pounds of fish a *year!*)

At about the same time, an Australian researcher who fed volunteers egg yolks and fish oil found that the blood cholesterol of the volunteers remained at healthy levels despite the cholesterol in the egg yolks.

What does this mean to you?

Fish oils are rich in highly unsaturated omega-3 fatty acids which appear to prevent your blood platelets from sticking together to form dangerous clots. Extensive studies reveal that the omega-3 fatty acids found in oily fish seem to block the body's production of LDL cholesterol. These studies also show omega-3 fatty acids lower plasma triglycerides, and artery-clogging blood fats. That is the good news. The bad news is that fish oils don't appear to have a significant effect on lowering LDL cholesterol unless they are eaten in the context of a diet that conforms to U. S. Dietary Goals of 30% fat or less!

So, what about the fish oil supplements that are popular at health food stores? Despite the exciting evidence that fish oils may help prevent heart disease, the American Heart Association advises against taking the fish oil supplements. More recent studies show that although these products are often prescribed by physicians in the belief they may lower blood triglyceride levels (which are different than cholesterol levels), they do nothing to lower LDL production. In fact, fish oil supplements usually create vitamin imbalances and have been shown to adversely affect the way blood clots. These same researchers point to evidence that shows we get the best LDL lowering effect simply by eating fish two or three times a week. That is good news, because it fits right in with lowfat lifestyle goals.

The fish with the most omega-3 fatty acids are those we have traditionally avoided because they are higher in total fat. They are the fish that swim in cold ocean waters: salmon, mackerel, tuna and sardines. Some other high protein foods also contain omega-3 oils, but these foods are not believed to be as efficient at decreasing LDL levels.

When you choose to eat these "higher fat" fish, be sure you poach, bake, steam or grill them. Frying fish can actually dilute any beneficial results that may occur from eating them. Avoid covering fish with high fat sauces. And remember, despite these new studies, the best way to keep your triglycerides and cholesterol levels down is to move back to basics. Cut down the *total* fat in your diet!

FISH with OMEGA-3 OILS   (listed high to low)

Chinook salmon
Atlantic mackerel
Bluefin tuna
Rainbow trout
Snow crab
Atlantic herring
Swordfish

Red snapper
Halibut
Pacific whiting
Haddock
Flounder
Sole

OTHER FOODS with OMEGA-3 OILS

Walnuts
Soybeans
Oats
Wheat germ

Navy beans
Pinto beans
Lima beans
Dried peas

REMEMBER: No matter how healthy, all oils are 100% fat!

LIFE
    is a process...we are ever changing
        and growing
            and learning
                and knowing that...

LIFE
    is a process...

GETTING THE
NUMBERS STRAIGHT

Americans are getting smart. They like making wise choices in their lives, including knowing more about the food they eat. Having learned that the amount of fat in an individual food and in our total diet contributes significantly to our health and our levels of body fat, most people want to know how much fat is in the food they eat. So, I was not surprised when Ken arrived at my office with five food packages and said, "You told me food providers are beginning to respond to consumer requests for more package information. These packages contain the information that is required on labels. They also highlight information that tells how many grams of carbohydrate, fat, protein and percentage of U. S. Recommended Daily Allowances are present in one serving of the food. How can I use this information to compute the calories of fat in each serving of food, or the percent of fat in the food itself? And how can I tell where it falls in the context of the 20% weight loss plan we have outlined? In other words, Ronda, is this label of any practical use to me?"

Ken had good reason to be confused. The supposedly helpful package information on some products does not go far enough. But with a few math tools you can use this information to compute the calories of fat in each serving of the food, the percent fat of the food and where that food falls in the context of a 30 percent or less fat diet.

CONVERSION OF GRAMS TO CALORIES

First learn how to convert grams of food to calories of food. To do so you need to know that:

- a gram of protein contains 4 calories
- a gram of carbohydrate contains 4 calories
- a gram of fat contains 9 calories

To convert grams of food to calories of food multiply the number of grams by the calories per gram. For example:

**To convert 7 grams of protein to calories,
7 grams x 4 calories per gram = 28 calories of protein.**

**To convert 6 grams of carbohydrate to calories,
6 grams x 4 calories per gram = 24 calories of carbohydrate.**

**To convert 5 grams of fat to calories,
5 grams x 9 calories per gram = 45 calories of fat.**

Working it out:
Suppose you have a label for Wheat Nuts snack. It has:
  4 grams of protein,
  5 grams of carbohydrate,
  8 grams of fat.

To convert these to calories of protein, carbohydrate and fat:

**4 grams protein x 4 calories per gram protein
= 16 calories of protein**

**5 grams carbohydrate x 4 calories per carbohydrate
= 20 calories carbohydrate**

8 grams fat x 9 calories per gram fat = 72 calories of fat

Now you try it:
A popular brand of cereal has:
>   2 grams of protein,
>   19 grams of carbohydrate,
>   5 grams of fat.

How many calories of protein?
How many of calories of carbohydrate?
How many calories of fat?

CALCULATIONS HERE:

(The answer is 8 protein, 76 carbohydrate and 45 of fat.)

COMPUTING THE PERCENT OF FAT IN THE FOOD
To compute the percentage of fat calories in the food you
need to know the total number of fat calories (step one) and
the total number of calories per serving. This latter information will be on the food package. Use the following formula:

$$\frac{\text{total number of fat calories}}{\text{total calories}} \times 100 = \text{\% of fat calories}$$

WORKING IT OUT
Suppose you have a package of lowfat yogurt. The label
provides you with the following nutrition information:

Serving size	8 oz.
Servings per container	1
Calories per serving	240
Protein	x grams
Carbohydrate	x grams
Fat	4 grams

To convert the grams of fat to calories of fat, multiply the grams of fat (4) by 9 (the number of calories in a gram of fat)

4 X 9 = 36 total fat calories

To compute the percent of fat of this yogurt divide the fat calories (36) by the total calories per serving (240).

$$\frac{36 \text{ fat calories}}{240 \text{ total calories}} \times 100 = 15\% \text{ fat.}$$

This yogurt is 15% fat.

The American Heart Association, American Dietetic Association and American Cancer Society agree that a 25-30 percent fat diet is the goal for optimum health. In my experience, a 20 percent fat diet will result in the use of stored body fat for muscle fuel and, eventually, a loss of weight as body fat for most people. If you are very overfat, at coronary risk or have yo-yo dieted for a long period of time, you may need to cut the percentage to as low as 10-15 percent of your total calories to see the changes you desire. But even if you are very fit, 25-30 percent is the maximum amount of fat you should eat every day. Where does that fit into your diet plan?

COMPUTING THE GRAMS OF FAT IN YOUR DIET
Suppose you are an active male, have no fat to lose, and you eat a balanced and varied diet of about 2400 calories a day. If an optimum diet is 25 percent fat:

2400 calories x .25 = 600 calories.

Since there are 9 calories in a gram of fat, you divide the 600 calories by 9 to determine the maximum number of grams of fat that make up a 25 percent fat diet.

$$\frac{600 \text{ calories}}{9 \text{ calories per gram}} = 67 \text{ grams of fat}$$

On the other hand, suppose you are a woman who is overfat and you want to reduce your calorie intake to about 1500 calories. You plan to exercise and eat a 20 percent fat diet. How many grams of fat is that?

1500 x .20 = 300 calories of fat

Since there are 9 calories in a gram of fat you can divide the 300 calories by 9 calories per gram to determine the maximum number of grams of fat that make up a 20% fat diet.

$$\frac{\textbf{300 calories}}{\textbf{9 calories per gram}} = \textbf{33 grams of fat}$$

The important thing to remember as you calculate the allowable grams of fat in your diet is that this "allotted" fat is in the context of *total* calories. If you are going to monitor grams of fat intake you *must* also monitor *total* food intake to be sure you are eating a balanced and varied diet that has sufficient calories. Resources like The Food Book and Food Values of Commonly Used Foods by Pennington and Church can help you determine the fat and calorie content of foods.

Although you may not enjoy recording your food intake, it is important to find and use a system that you are willing to maintain throughout the early days of lifestyle change. Soon you will be able to monitor food intake mentally. In addition to the books I referred to above, a variety of professional systems and computerized diet analysis programs in most communities provide this service for a fee. Registered dietitians are excellent resources for diet analysis. If you do not have access to a computerized diet analysis program to make these computations I suggest the diet analysis concept described by Covert Bailey in The Fit-Or-Fat Target Diet.

Do not make the mistake Carolyn made after she heard me explain this idea. She calculated how many grams of fat she could eat per day but that was *all* she monitored. When she didn't lose weight I suggested we review her diet records together. Carolyn was eating her allotted amount of fat but very little carbohydrate and protein to round out her diet. It was 62% fat. When she added more carbohydrate and non-fat protein her diet dropped back to a 20% fat level and the pounds started coming off slowly.

COMPUTING THE PERCENT OF FAT IN YOUR DIET
If you know the total fat calories (grams of fat x 9) and total food calories (using calorie counting guides, diet analysis sheets or professional assistance) here is how you can determine the percent of fat in your diet.

$$\frac{\text{total number of fat calories}}{\text{total calories in the diet}} = \text{\% of fat calories}$$

Check out your own refrigerator and cupboard. Are your packaged foods high or low in fat? Before you throw out all your "old" food choices, remember: The *total* fat and/or recommended maximum grams of fat in the diet is the ultimate goal of any weight loss or weight maintenance program. If you choose to eat a high fat food, balance it with a low fat food, so the *average* is in accordance with your personal goals. You want a *balance* between the high fat food you purchased before you learned this skill and the low fat food you can now find on the supermarket shelves-because you are better informed.

Weight management is much easier once you have the tools to make wise choices! After you have computed calories of fat and percentage of fat from 5-10 labels you will be a smart shopper and well on your way to knowing how to measure fat.

IT'S ALL
ON THE LABEL

Charlotte was assuming responsibilities for personal training services at a local health club. In addition to monitoring
the exercise of their clients, the trainers planned to provide
the bites of knowledge that could help them choose foods
more wisely. They wanted to include information that could
contribute to smarter supermarket shopping habits. They
asked me where they should begin.

"Labels," I said. "Start by reading labels on food packages."

Charlotte was surprised. "Why read labels?" she asked.
"Because they contain information that can help you get the
most out of your food dollar." I replied.

We take food labels for granted. On close examination they
can look pretty complicated–unless you have some savvy
about what kind of information is there, why it is there and
what it really means.

Food labels are regulated by the Food and Drug Administra-

tion. By law all food labels must contain:
  *the name of the product
  *the quantity of the product in the package
  *the ingredients in the food— listed by weight, not volume
  *the name and place of business where you may write for additional information
  *any required warnings. For example, foods containing saccharin must include the warning, "Use of this product may be hazardous to your health."

Any time a nutrition claim is made or a nutrient is added to a food the label must also show "nutrition information". This additional information includes:
  *the number of servings per package or container
  *the serving size on which the nutrition information (including calories per serving) is based
  *the calories and grams of protein fat and carbohydrate and the U. S. Recommended Daily Allowances for what are known as "leader nutrients."

Some food packages contain additional information that is considered optional. It usually includes milligrams of cholesterol per serving, types of fats and types of carbohydrates, and sodium content. All of this label information is important and you will read more about it in subsequent chapters of this book.

As I continued talking to Charlotte's group I suggested they be aware that consumers are prey for manufacturers who operate with the knowledge that labels can't lie but liars can write labels.

Charlotte was one step ahead of me. "You still haven't mentioned the descriptive terms on labels, she said. "

"You're right," I agreed. "Most descriptive terms used on labels are placed there with an eye toward the psychological issues that make a product more or less attractive to the buyer." Since many of these terms are *not* regulated by the Food and Drug Administration I suggested we review the more common ones found on food packages.

• ENRICHED–When a food is processed it loses some of it's nutrients. An enriched food has some of these nutrients re-added. Breads and cereals are usually enriched.

• FORTIFIED–If a nutrient has been added to a food that it does not contain naturally, the food has been fortified. For example milk is fortified with Vitamin D and some orange juice is now fortified with calcium.

• REDUCED CALORIE–A product that has at least 1/3 less calories than the food it replaces can be labeled reduced calorie. Good examples include lower in fat mayonnaise or salad dressings.

• IMITATION–These foods bear no chemical or nutritional resemblance to the foods they imitate. Some examples include imitation low cholesterol egg products and imitation jam.

• LOW CALORIE–A food labeled low calorie can have no more than 40 calories per serving or 0.4 calories per gram.

• SUGAR FREE–Beware of this one. It only means it contains no sucrose. There are lots of other sweeteners on the market that are not wise choices when you are thinking about reducing the sugar content of your diet . (see page 47.)

• LITE or LIGHT–There are no regulations for the use of the word "light." It can mean light in calories, light in color or light in weight. Buyer beware!

• NATURAL–This one is really tricky. *Anything* can be labeled natural. Just because something is natural doesn't mean it is good for you. For example, bacteria and viruses are natural.

• LOW CHOLESTEROL–The use of this term does not mean low fat or low in saturated fats. It just means low in cholesterol.

• LOW FAT–The use of the words "low fat" is not regulated by law, but is generally agreed to be less than 25% calories as fat.

• SALT FREE or NO SALT–This means no more than 5

milligrams of sodium chloride. But beware: sodium chloride, table salt, is only one of many sodium compounds in food (i.e., sodium bicarbonate, monosodium glutamate). (See page 55).

• **LOW SODIUM**–A food labeled "low sodium" must have 140 milligrams or less per serving.

• **VERY LOW SODIUM**–A food labeled "very low sodium" must have 35 milligrams or less per serving.

• **ORGANIC**-The word "organic" means "containing carbon." All living substances (plants and animals) contain carbon. This makes almost all our food organic! In health food stores "organic" usually refers to the method of farming used to produce the food in which no pesticides, herbicides, or chemical fertilizers are used.

• **DIETETIC**–Any food can be labeled dietetic if it contains even one less calorie than the normal food. Many dietetic candies are no lower in fat than regular candies.

ADDED FIBER–15-25 grams of dietary fiber is suggested for prevention of colon cancer. Crude fiber doesn't count.

The trainers agreed that when they purchase food they want the best their money can buy. If the food label is a legal contract between the food manufacturer and the buyer, understanding the terms that describe food is important in assuring their part of the "deal." They chatted among themselves and came up with their own nutrition education slogan, "supermarket beware." I knew their clients would soon agree.

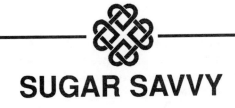

SUGAR SAVVY

Have you seen the new statistics that say that individual sugar consumption in the U. S. has dropped to about 65 pounds per person in the last few years. Not true. The average American eats about 130 pounds of "sugar" each year. That is the equivalent of 40 teaspoons per day (600 calories). The discrepancy is a matter of semantics. The reason the marketing world can get away with those kind of "inaccuracies" is because there is more than one way to describe "sugar".

We eat most sugar as a refined product hidden in processed foods we buy for convenience. There are a lot of other ways to describe these empty calories besides the cane sugar we know as white table sugar or sucrose originally refined by the Persians in 600 A. D.

The increase in diabetes and syndromes often described as hypoglycemia, or "low blood sugar" are in direct proportion to the increase, not a decrease, in the amount of sugar we eat. There is also evidence to support a link between sugar and, depression, eating disorders and substance addictions. This has resulted in an effort by savvy entrepeneurs to develop and encourage our use of other sweetening agents. These new products have been incorporated into many of the packaged foods you buy. Buyers, beware! Advertising and promotion "specialists" often take advantage of this change and label products "sugar free" in the hope you will think they are better choices. They are not. On page 41 you learned the words "sugar free" only mean there is no sucrose or white refined table sugar in the food. Until all the information is in, avoiding too much sugar–no matter what it is called–is going to help you conform to the lifestyle that health promotion professionals encourage you to adopt.

To help get you started here is a list of some sugar saturated foods so lacking in nutrition they don't deserve to be called foods. They include:

jams	soft drinks
jellies	noodle mix
preserves	sugar cereals
desserts	cocoa mix
candy bars	sherbet
ice cream	whiskey mixes

Would you believe the following foods have these amounts of sugar?

fudge, 5 tsp.	glazed donut, 6 tsp.
can cola, 9 tsp.	4 oz. tang, 16 tsp.
Big Gulp, 25 tsp.	6 oz. yogurt, 5 tsp.
one cup cider, 6 tsp.	pkg. noodle mix 9 tsp.
2 fig bars, 10 tsp.	

They do.

I emphasize getting the fat out of the diet, but the decreased intake of empty sugar calories is also important when you are improving your eating habits. You will need some savvy about label reading if you are going to beat the advertising manipulators. Here are the names of some common substitutes for "sugar" currently available in processed foods:

FRUCTOSE is supposedly sweeter than sucrose so "you don't need to use as much". That is true only if it is cold. True, fructose does not raise blood sugar levels as much as dextrose and sucrose do, so it's less of a problem for diabetics. But fructose is empty of nutritional calories nonetheless and it causes gastrointestinal disturbances in many individuals. **BROWN SUGAR**, at 17 calories per teaspoon, is nutritionally equivalent to white sugar. It is made by adding a little molasses (made from sugar) to white sugar.

CORN SYRUP is made when corn starch is broken down by acids, resulting in a clear, somewhat sweet liquid. It is a sugar.

MOLASSES is a thick, dark syrup which is a by-product of table sugar made from sugar cane.

HONEY is a popular sugar substitute because it's slightly sweeter than sugar, so people believe they are using less sweetener and getting less calories.That is not true. Honey has 22 calories per teaspoon. Sugar has 16 calories per teaspoon. Using honey as a substitute for sugar in a recipe *does not* save calories. Honey enthusiasts also encourage its use because it "has vitamins in it" and because "it is made by the little bees, so it is natural". There is no nutritional advantage to using honey instead of sugar. Honey does contain trace calcium, iron, and phosphorus. However, these nutrients are more efficiently obtained from milk and eggs. And.....

It takes:	To get the equivalent of:
296 tbsp. honey (18,944 calories)	**calcium from 1 cup skim milk** (88 calories)
162 tbsp. honey (10,368 calories)	**iron from 3 oz. liver** (234 calories)
103 tbsp. honey (6592 calories)	**phosphorus from 1 egg** (82 calories)
24 tbsp. honey	**potassium in an orange.**

I could go on and on, but the bottom line is: Sugars can be disguised on package labels when they are called:

corn syrup	dextrose
fructose	hexitol
glucose	invert sugar
mannitol	molasses
saccharin	sorbitol
sucrose	refined
maltose	corn sweetener
dextrin	cane
levulose	honey
xylitol	maple syrup
brown sugar	turbinado sugar
"raw" sugar	confectioner's sugar

Next time you go to the store, pick up the packaged goods you are used to throwing in your basket unconsciously and see if they contain more than one kind of sugar. Then think about it. Is it really the best choice for your palate and your family's long term health? And, beware!

BULKING UP

Grandma called it roughage. When incorporated into weight loss products it's called bulk. It is also known as a laxative. The American Cancer Society says it can prevent cancer and cardiologists tell us that it can help protect against heart disease. What is this magic ingredient? It's fiber.

Fiber is a general term for a material found in most plants that cannot be digested by human beings. When I talk about it during a lecture I say the primary virtue of fiber is that it gives us something for nothing. I am talking about satiety, but before I can explain what I mean there is usually a lot of tittering and giggling. That's because most people immediately think of the unpleasant side effect of a high fiber diet: flatulence. Or as the kids say, (intestinal) gaaaaaasssss.

Well, it's time to throw caution to the wind and find out what fiber is all about.

In the last chapter we talked about sugars or carbohydrates. The scientific name for a carbohydrate is a saccharide.

Carbohydrates are either monosaccharides, disaccharides or polysaccharides. At the risk of being to simplistic let us say a monosaccharide looks like this:

When two monosaccharides are linked together they form a disaccharide, which might look like this:

If more than two disaccharides are linked it is called a polysaccharide, which might look like this:

♦ - ♦ - ♦

Or, suppose the polysaccharides linked up with one another. For awhile they might continue on a straight line like this:

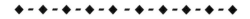

But, I like to think of polysaccharides as being playful. After a bunch of them string themselves together they like to start crossing lines with one another, connecting with more than one or two other saccharides much like the game children play where they hold hands then start stepping over one another's arms. In this case the configuration of the saccharides becomes more complex and might look something like this:

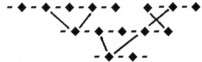

These very big polysaccharides are called complex carbohydrates because they are linked together in such a complex "web" that they cannot be broken apart during digestion. Instead they pass through your digestive system unchanged.

Fiber is a *very* complex carbohydrate. Fiber yields no calories but makes you feel full when it absorbs many times its weight in water in the small intestines. This same water absorbing property has a stool softening effect making it easier for you to eliminate body wastes. Fiber also acts as a binder for food and as scrubbers for your large intestines. These properties of fiber keep your food moving quickly through your digestive tract. That may decrease the exposure time to naturally occuring intestinal cancer causing agents as well as the ability to remove them.

For those of us interested in managing our weight, these plant-based foods that are high in fiber are also lower in calories than fat and cholesterol containing animal products. Since they are chewy they take longer to eat and their ability to absorb water makes us feel full longer than when we eat a low fiber diet.

Because fiber is not an essential nutrient there are no recommendations for how much or what kind we should eat. All health promotion specialists agree, however, that the American diet is too low in fiber. It just makes good sense to eat more of it. And remember, "life is a gas."

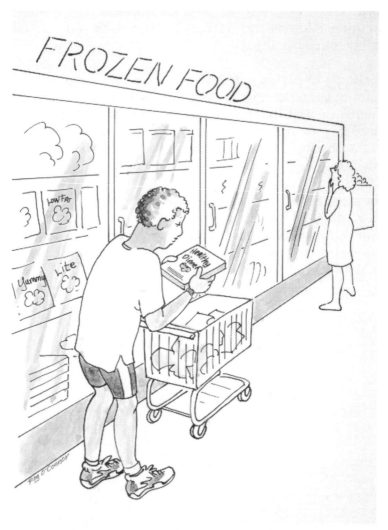

"Contains no sugar, salt, fat, cholesterol,
preservatives, artificial flavorings or taste."

ABOUT SODIUM

What do table, garlic, onion, celery and seasoned salt, monosodium glutamate, baking soda, saccharin, sodium nitrate, and sodium benzoate have in common? They are all "salts" and all are sources of sodium. Sodium is a naturally occuring mineral found in many foods including vegetables, fish, fresh meats, dairy products and eggs. Even water contains some sodium. Sodium and potassium maintain fluid balance in the body and help transmit electrical messages from nerves to muscles, so we need them. But how much is too much?

Adults need barely 200 miligrams of sodium per day. Recommendations are to limit our intake to one gram per day (1/2 teaspoon = 1 gram). However, most Americans eat two to three times that amount, mostly hidden as preservatives and additives that enhance flavor and preserve the processed foods we eat.

Have you ever experienced swollen hands or feet after eating a particularly salty meal? This is the result of shifts in fluids in the body when it tries to maintain the homeostasis or balanced pH necessary for good health. In fact, one of the more interesting syndromes sometimes seen in hospital emergency rooms is called "Chinese food syndrome". The patient is admitted with a severe headache, heart failure or other symptoms caused by a work overload placed on the heart. This overload is the result of an increase in interstitial fluid to keep pH balanced after you eat a very salty meal. The name resulted from observing many of these idiosyncratic reactions in people who had eaten lots of monosodium glutamate (MSG) served at Chinese restaurants.

We acquire our taste for salt, and most people who salt their food never think about tasting it before they use their salt shaker. Salt is one flavor enhancer that is easy to remove from the diet. You can decrease the amounts of salt added in any cooking, learn how to read labels on packaged food products to determine the amount of sodium in a serving and increase your savvy about using other seasonings that can replace salt. Purchase and cook more fresh foods. When I occasionally open a can of soup or a low calorie frozen dinner for a quick low fat meal I am appalled by the salty taste. I have lost my taste for salt. Most soups and packaged frozen foods contain almost a teaspoon of salt in a serving! That is more than is recommended we eat in a single day!

Medically, there continues to be considerable controversy as to whether too much MSG or any other sodium in the diet leads to high blood pressure due to the extra effort required of the heart to overcome this fluid retention overload. Until the verdict is in, cardiac risk patients are encouraged to restrict sodium by using the suggestions in the previous paragraph and using many of the low sodium or low salt products on the market. Some of the saltier foods to avoid include canned vegetables, tomato and vegetable juices, pickled products, preserved meats, bouillon, fast foods, chips and other snacks, soft drinks and soups–especially instant soup mixes.

I am always happy to find ways to help people make easy beginnings. Decreasing salt intake is one of them.

CAFFEINE
IS IT WORTH THE LIFT?

My former pharmacy and current health promotion careers continue to cross paths. Often in post-lecture discussions someone asks me about drugs and foods and moods, and we explore the possibility that all foods have the potential to be drugs. That is not far out of the stream of traditional thinking. And if someone asked me, "what is the most widely used drug in the world?" I'd say, "Caffeine". Each morning, millions of Americans, and people all over the world, stumble out of bed and head straight for the coffee or tea pot or pour a glass of their favorite cola beverage. Before the day ends more than 80 percent of us drink or eat the equivilent of two to three cups of caffeinated coffee. More coffee is consumed in the U. S than any other country in the world. Four out of five Americans have two to four cups every day, while twenty five percent qualify as true caffeine addicts by drinking more than five cups in a 24 hour period.

Caffeine has been around a long time. Chinese literature dated 2700 B. C. talks about its effects. In the U. S., until 1980 when scientific studies raised questions about its safety, caffeine was described by the Food and Drug Admnistration as "generally recognized as safe."

The jury is still out on the relative seriousness of the effects of caffeine intake. Although studies continue to disagree, all health educators generally agree that because caffeine is a drug it should be avoided or, at least, used in moderation.

Since there is a lot of true and false folklore about caffeine, here are some hard facts I compiled from official and non-official literature about this controversial substance.

Chemically, caffeine is one of a group of compounds called xanthines. It is a mild central nervous stimulant found in coffee, tea, cola beverages, chocolate and many prescription and nonprescription medicines, especially analgesics and cold remedies. It also doubles as a flavoring agent in baked goods, desserts and puddings; the slightly bitter flavor is used to balance the sweetness of the sugar in these products. In other words, unless you know what is in everything you put in your mouth, chances are you swallow some every day.

Your individual reaction to caffeine will be influenced by several factors including the amount you consume in relation to your body weight, your age, your emotional or nervous state and your individual tolerance or "threshold." When you realize how important these factors are it is easy to see how much more sensitive children are to caffeine "dosages" in food and drink that may be one-third to one-half the amount that affect an adult.

But is caffeine bad for you? It depends on who you talk to. Caffeine has been identified as a culprit in the development of cancer, heart disease and ulcers. It has been linked to birth defects and the painful, noncancerous cysts or lumps of fibrocystic breast disease. It has also been praised as an adjunct to headache medications, and for decreasing the wheeze of asthma by opening bronchial passages.

Because caffeine releases fatty acids into the blood stream it is used by athletes as a tool for improving performance in endurance exercise. This conserves more glycogen (stored muscle fuel from carbohydrates) that can be used later in the race, thereby increasing endurance. But, new studies show this effect is lost in people who use caffeine regularly. Despite a study that supported the more fat in blood theory, most physiologists believe the effect of caffeine on athletic performance is psychological instead of physiological.

Caffeine creates a state of wakefulness within 15 minutes after you swallow it and the effects last for two hours or more. Caffeine has also been proven to increase alertness, decrease fatigue, and suppress appetite. It is a mood booster, and a study at the Massachusetts Institute of Technology showed it can improve mental performance.

Caffeine acts as a diuretic (a drug that increases urine production) by decreasing the reabsorption of sodium and chloride into the blood from the tubes in the kidneys. People who want to get rid of excess body fluid seek this effect, but it can be dangerous on hot days or during long races when it may cause dehydration and gastric distress.

A personal experience with caffeine: When I was living in Lake Tahoe I was stunned when I was diagnosed as having a kidney stone. The doctor told me there is a much higher incidence of kidney stones at that 7500 foot elevation where the body dehydrates more quickly. When I had moved to Tahoe from sea level Portland, Oregon, I continued my habit of drinking caffeine laden diet cola; it had never occurred to me how important it was to replace and increase my fluid intake to compensate for the dehydrating combination of diuretic and altitude. I've subsequently wondered if people who travel regularly in the dry cabins of airplanes, where they refresh and entertain themselves with diet cokes and other dehydrating drinks, are aware of the consequences to their bodies. I also wonder how many kidney stones or other dehydrative symptoms (dry skin, dandruff, weak muscles and cramps) are caused by this combination of drug and environment.

When you eat or drink substances containing caffeine the speed with which it gets into your blood stream is dependent on the amount of food in your stomach. Once caffeine enters your blood it increases your heart rate, promotes secretion of stomach acid, speeds up urine production, dilates some blood vessels and constricts others. If you have ever experienced "coffee nerves" you know how caffeine can cause trembling, depression, diarrhea, loss of appetite, nervousness, and chronic muscle tension. Excessive intake, about 1,000 milligrams a day (the equivalent of ten cups of coffee), leads to extreme restlessness, insomnia, headaches, heart palpitations, gastrointestinal complaints and in some susceptible people, panic attacks.

Caffeine also effects the electrical system of the heart; if you have heart trouble and high blood pressure, avoid coffee.

A study in Norway, a high coffee consuming population, suggests that people who drink one to four cups of coffee a day increase their blood cholesterol levels by five percent. If they drink five to eight cups per day it was elevated nine percent, and nine or more cups of coffee per day raised cholesterol levels 12 percent higher than those of non-drinkers.

Women who drink large amounts of beverages containing caffeine are seven times more likely to report moderate to severe pre-menstrual syndrome (PMS) symptoms than those who do not consume caffeine.

Caffeine has been reported by many medical researchers to aggravate pain and fluid retention in fibrocystic (lumpy breasts) conditions. One study showed that eliminating caffeine from the diet brought extraordinary relief from fibrocystic disease (I participated in this one and concur). Another study reported no effect.

Caffeine affects some people more than others. Although it hasn't been shown to be as physiologically addictive as "hard" drugs such as cocaine or opium, caffeine withdrawal can trigger severe headaches, jitters, irritability, sleepiness and reduced alertness. And as it does in response to most addictive substances, the body becomes more and more used to the drug; people who use caffeine for its stimulant quantities need more and more. If you are a smoker this tolerance builds more easily.

The addictive quality of caffeine can provide a moral dilemma for athletes subject to guidelines for blood "doping". Caffeine is not an illegal substance and most people "use" it every day. Pharmacologically it is considered a drug at levels of above 4 milligrams per kilogram of body weight. To date, although the use of caffeine is not endorsed, there is no regulating athletic organization that tests athletes or penalizes them for its use.

How much of this confusing drug is in our daily food and drink? Examine this chart which was compiled from a variety of sources (which leads to a variety of data).

Source	Milligrams of Caffeine
*Coffee (5 oz. cup)	115
Drip method	80
Percolated	65
Instant	
Decaffeinated, brewed	3
Decaffeinated, instant	2
*Tea (5 oz. cup)	40
Brewed, domestic	60
Brewed, imported	30
Green	30
Instant	
Iced (12 oz. glass)	70
Canned Iced	29

Chocolate	
Chocolate milk (8 oz. glass)	5-10
Dark chocolate, semisweet (2 oz.)	20
Chocolate bar (2 oz.)	30
Milk chocolate (1 oz.)	6
Cocoa (5 oz. cup)	50

Soft drinks (12 oz. can)	
Diet Mr. Pibb	59
Mountain Dew	54
Mello Yellow	52
Tab	46
Coca-Cola	46
Diet Coke	46
Shasta Cola	44
Sunkist Orange	42
Dr. Pepper & Sugar Free Dr. Pepper	41
Pepsi-Cola	38
Diet Pepsi	36
RC Cola	36
Diet Rite	36

There is no caffeine in root beer, ginger ale, 7-up like drinks, decaffeinated cola, tonic water, club soda or seltzer.
* The amount of caffeine can vary greatly, depending on how long the beverage is brewed.

One study I reviewed said that caffeine has been added to more than 1,000 non-prescription medications including diet pills, stay-awake pills, cold tablets and headache and allergy remedies, but here are some of the most common:.

Nonprescription drugs (per tablet)

APC (analgesic)	32
Anacin & Anacin Maximum Strength (analgesic)	32
Aqua-Ban (diuretic)	100
Caffedrine (stimulant)	200
Cope (analgesic)	32
Coryban-D (cold remedy)	30
Dexatrim (weight management)	200
Dietac (weight management)	200
Dristan (cold remedy)	32
Empirin Compound (analgesic)	32
Excedrin (analgesic)	65
Midol (analgesic)	32
No Doz (stimulant)	200
Permethene H2 Off (diuretic)	200
Pre-Mens (diuretic)	66
Pre-Mens Forte (diuretic)	100
Prolamine (weight management)	140
Triaminicin (cold remedy)	30
Vanquish (analgesic)	33
Vivarin (stimulant)	200

There is no caffeine in plain aspirin. The caffeine in most cold medications is there to counteract the sleepiness caused by the antihistamines in the medication.

Prescription drugs (per capsule)

Cafergot (for migraine headaches; constricts blood vessels)	100
Cafermine (for migraine headaches; constricts blood vessels)	100
Cafetrate (for migraine headaches; constricts blood vessels)	100
Darvon Compund-65 (painkiller)	32
Esgic (for tension headaches)	40
Fiorinal (for tension headache)	40
Migral (for migraine headaches; constricts blood vessels)	100
Synalgos-DC (strong analgesic)	30

AND when you mix caffeine and other substances:	Effect:
Oral Contraceptives	increases caffeine effect
MAO Inhibitors (anti depressants)	increases blood pressure
Thyroid hormones	increases drug effect
Isoniazid	increases drug effect
Alcohol	decreases intoxication
Mother's milk	drug enters milk
Tagamet (ulcer medication	increases caffeine effect
Tranquilizers, sleeping pills	decreases drug effect
Cigarettes	decreases caffeine effect
Cocaine	dangerous over-stimulation
Marijuana	increases effect of both, and increases heart rate

The most common caffeine withdrawal symptom is a headache that begins as early as 16 hours or as late as two weeks after the last "dose". Withdrawal headaches often hang on for several days. If you don't withdraw gradually from the use of caffeine the headache can be severe. The irony is that caffeine is added to analgesics for the treatment of headaches because it reduces tension in blood vessels in the brain. It also relieves the muscle tension caused by headaches by increasing blood flow to muscle cells. However, the drug is useful only for headaches caused by high blood pressure. (Migraine headaches fall into this category). Caffeine's use in combination with aspirin and phenacetin for other kinds of headaches is highly questionable. Since two to three cups of coffee can raise blood pressure by 14 percent (with the effect wearing off as the body adapts to the caffeine) you can see how headaches can be part of a vicious addictive cycle.

The effects of caffeine withdrawal include headache, irritability, and drowsiness. To avoid these withdrawal effects taper your intake of foods, beverages and medications that contain caffeine over a one month period. For example, begin by lowering the amount of caffeine released in coffee by shortening the brewing time or by mixing caffeine containing coffee with de-caf. Drugs should be discontinued under a doctors care.

Like many other mood altering foods caffeine does not have to meet any FDA or U. S. Department of Agriculture standards. If it did, caffeine would probably not be available, except by prescription. Because it is a drug, caffeine should be avoided or, (at least) used in moderation. If you choose to use caffeine, avoid it after mid-afternoon. Eat a balanced and varied diet, exercise regularly, and be sure you get the amount of sleep you need.

That is the best key to awakening to normal stimulation and remaining drug-free. Like all products, processes and people we use to change who we really are, there is a fine line between enjoying, using and becoming addicted to what the world puts in front of us. And those decisions are up to us!

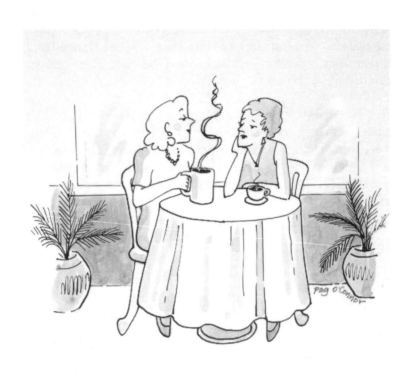

"I'm down to one cup of coffee a day."

LET'S DINE OUT

"I don't cook," Jack told me. I eat out three times a day so what you've told me about shopping and cooking doesn't apply for me."

"Eating out" is such an integral part of American life these days that even if you don't eat out as often as Jack does it is important for you to acquire some savvy about how to maintain a lowfat lifestyle in those situations which may challenge your best eating interests. Whether you are "on the road", making a quick stop between errands or eating out for social pleasure, here are some tips that can help you meet this challenge in a sometimes alien environment.

Try dividing your eating out experiences into two kinds–those where the outing is a convenience and those where the outing is a special occasion. Meals "on the go" and meals where you need to "take care of business", whether your own or with others, fit into the first category. A special occasion can be around an event, with loved ones or as a treat for yourself.

Consider letting go of your judgement as to whether menu choices are good or bad. That black and white attitude can predispose you to failure. Instead, look at food as wiser and poorer choices. Within the framework of a balanced and varied low fat, low sugar, high fiber diet even a fatty and sugary splurge can be a wise choice if it will satisfy you emotionally as well as physically. The important issue is to notice where you are and what you want, explore your options and make the choice that elevates your self esteem.

Monitoring your diet is another tool that can assure your choices fit into a total eating plan. For example, I have learned that recording my daily food intake and noticing my moods when I choose to eat has been the most significant factor contributing to my client's and my own success with long term weight management. If you don't monitor your daily fat, sugar and fiber intake by recording your food on a daily basis, commit to do so during those periods when you will be in situations that prevent you from fixing your own meals. (I like the diet analysis method described by Covert Bailey in <u>Fit or Fat Target Diet</u>). This kind of record keeping has helped me avoid guilt about any splurging I might do. It also helps me become aware of the kind of eating I am doing and to "save " fat calories for an upcoming meal. Then I can comfortably take part, even celebrate, as I enjoy foods I don't eat on a regular basis. As a result of this new technique to take care of myself, dining out is no longer sabotaging to my new way of eating.

In addition, an understanding of the words and phrases that describe food has helped me make prudent choices and remain "on target" in a restaurant.

The traditional advice about ordering broiled, steamed or boiled poultry or fish rather than "greasy" (not red) meat still applies. In addition, food described in the following manner is an indication it is prepared with very little fat:
Steamed: To cook in steam in a pressure cooker, deep well cooker, double boiler or a steamer made by fitting a rack in

a pan with a tight cover. A small amount of boiling water is used.

Broiled: To cook with dry heat, usually in a broiler or over coals (quick, direct heat).

Toasted: To prepare with dry heat in a toaster or oven.

Poached: To cook in hot liquid, being careful that the food holds its shape.

Seared: To brown very quickly by intense heat.

Braised: To brown in a small amount of hot fat, then add a small amount of liquid and cook slowly in a tightly covered utensil on a range or in an oven.

Stewed: To simmer slowly in a small amount of liquid for a long time.

Roasted: To cook slowly in a covered pan (dry heat cooking).

Grilled: If charcoaled or cooked over an open flame it is low fat-in some restaurants grilling means cooking on greasy flat top ranges.

Other ways of preparing foods with little or no fat include: **Garden fresh, In its own juice, Dry broiled, In lemon juice, Pickled, In tomato sauce or With cocktail sauce.**

These terms will help alert you to high fat food preparation:

Buttery	Escalloped	Bernaise
Au Gratin	Fried	French Fried
Prime	White Sauce	Hash
In Butter Sauce	Crispy	Pan Fried
Buttered	Marinated	In Gravy
Sauteed	Creamed	Marbled
Creamy	Hollandaise	A La Mode
In Cream Sauce	Basted	Bisque
Parmesan	Deep Fried	In Cheese Sauce

Here are a few pointers to help you make wise selections when dining out:

"Low calorie" and/or "low cholesterol" does not necessarily mean low fat. Cholesterol is just one kind of fat and low cholesterol menus usually indicate a choice of vegetable fat over animal fat in food preparation.

Be aware that low calorie recipes may have reduced calories but those that are there may be high in fat.

Don't hesitate to ask your waiter how your food is prepared or to inquire about the availability of foods that you may not see on the menu. For example, when a main dish includes a baked potato as a side dish I can usually get a baked potato and a salad with dressing on the side.

Be specific about what you do and do not want.

When possible, order a la carte. You will have more dishes and less food.

If you know where you are going to eat and what you would like to order, plan the remainder of your daily intake in a way that assures you will get all the nutrients you need.

If you find yourself noshing on chips or stuffing yourself with bread or rolls, ask that they be removed from the table.

Ask that your order be prepared with special care for eliminating fat.

Avoid butter, shortenings, margarine, mayonnaise, cream sauces, fried and breaded dishes and sauces and other foods that are high in fat.

Ask that your salad be served with the dressing "on the side". Then instead of pouring it over the salad, dip your fork into the dressing before each bite, then pick up the food. The combination of the metallic tines of the fork, the tangy salad dressing and the food hitting the tip of your tongue will more than make up for gobs of fatty dressing.

Without looking at the menu say, "I'll have a soup and a sandwich."

When fresh vegetables are available ask that they be steamed and served without sauces or butter.

If you have a choice between rice pilaf, french fries or a baked potato, take the potato without any toppings. When it arrives use your salad, other vegetables or juices from your meat or fish as a condiment.

Consider ordering several appetizers or vegetables or salads *instead* of a meal.

Choose foods that require you to work while you eat (crab, crayfish). It will keep you busy and you will eat less.

If you go to an all-you-can-eat buffet, stick to the foods that *satisfy* you. This is a place to *taste* foods, not to get the most for your money.

Delicatessen, health and gourmet food restaurants may have a lot of eye and psychological appeal but these foods are always high in fat. Choose them only on special occasions.

Be aware of what you want to eat (based on your own internal cues) rather than taking cues from what you see on the carefully designed menu in a restaurant where desserts may be prominently displayed.

Since alcohol is known to lower inhibitions around sensible food choices later in a meal, consider drinking soda or mineral water instead of an alcoholic beverage. If you enjoy wine with your meal, alternate each glass with one of water, mineral water, or diet soda.

Savor your food by eating as slowly as possible.

Pay attention to your appetite and stop eating when you feel full.

Avoid the temptation to eat everything that is put in front of you. It is not only okay but savvy to take part of your serving home for later.

Choose restaurants with a varied menu that offers alternatives that appeal to you.

If you know you will go to a restaurant often, ask the waiter if you can keep a copy of the menu to help you plan your pre-restaurant daily intake.

Ask that your plate be removed from the table before it's empty-if you are satisfied.

One of my biggest treats is room service when I am staying in a hotel. I order as many fresh steamed vegetables as I can get, and if I need more, add a salad. (P. S. It often costs less than a whole meal!)

Remember you can eat anything on the menu, especially if your body wants it.

My friend Carla Mulligan has a bizarre way of disciplining herself when unrequested, high fat foods are served to her. She immediately covers them with a heavy layer of salt! It is a sight to watch-she's found a successful way to make otherwise seductive foods unedible.

Foods that are a part of a lowfat lifestyle are available in most restaurants. Here is a list of selections to help you when you eat out!

APPETIZERS

Okay Selections	Selections of Concern
Radishes	Olives
Corn tortillas/Salsa	Cream soups
Carrots	Nuts
Fresh mushrooms	Cheese plates
Celery	Deep-fried anything
Salads (see salads)	
Fruit cup	
Broth-based soups	
Juice	
Shrimp/crab cocktail	

SALADS

Okay Selections	Selections of Concern
Tossed green	Cheddar cheese
Pickled beets	Swiss cheese
Fruit plate	Waldorf
Coleslaw (careful!)	Avocados
Jello	Olives
Three bean	German potato
Cucumber	Anything mayonnaise-based
Vegetable	Anything sour cream-based
Relish dish	
Chef's	
Cottage cheese	

SALADS, cont.

Okay Selections

Potato (careful again!)
Carrot-raisin
Cobb
Fresh fruit
Pasta

Remember. The dangerous part of most salads is the dressing! When you choose a salad with an oil or sour cream based dressing (like three bean or pasta) put it on top of your "greens" or mix it with other salad ingredients and don't use salad dressing.

SOUPS

Okay Selections	Selections of Concern
Chicken noodle	New England clam chowder
Vegetable	Cream soups
Barley	Bisques
French onion (no cheese)	
Tomato	
Minestrone	
Bouillabaisse	
Gazpacho	
Manhattan clam chowder	
Split Pea	
Any broth based soup	

ENTREES

(Remember, a serving size of meat is 3-4 ounces and of fish 4-5 ounces.)

Okay Selections

Fish-baked, broiled or poached
Spaghetti with tomato sauce
Cornish game hen (no skin)
Roast turkey
Baked ham
Roast lamb
Broiled or baked chicken (no skin)

Okay Selections

Shish kabob
Pot roast (plain)
Plain shellfish
Flank
Most Chinese dishes
Sirloin (trim the fat)
Tenderloin
Ground Sirloin or other extra lean ground meat
Whole wheat pizza with shellfish, fresh vegetables and skim milk cheese

---

Selections of Concern

Meatloaf
Whole milk cheese pizza or with sausage or with pepperoni
Chili con carne
Seafood au gratin
Creamed casseroles
Any breaded or fried entree
Burrito
Most cheese dishes
Pork and beans
Fried foods
Duck
Prime rib
Goose
Spareribs

Once In A While

Broiled pork chop
T-Bone steak
Porterhouse steak

SAUCES AND TOPPINGS (Try to avoid all or use sparingly.)

Tartar sauce	Gravy	Salad dressings
Margarine	Cream sauce	Hard sauce
Butter	Cheese sauce	Hollandaise
Mayonnaise	Sour cream	Whipped cream

Refer to the Quick Start List on page 22 of this book for a list of empty calorie foods that should be avoided whenever possible!

BEVERAGES

Okay Selections	Selections of Concern
Non-fat milk	Milkshakes
Tea	Whole milk
Buttermilk	Hot chocolate
Fruit juice	
Coffee	
Diet carbonated beverages	
Sparkling mineral water	
Lemonade, light on sugar	

BREAKFAST SELECTIONS

Okay Selections	Selections of Concern
Cottage cheese	Butter
English muffin	Tator Tots/hash browns
Bagel	Bacon
Dry Toast	Sausage
Lean Ham	Donuts
Poached eggs (2-3/week)	Danish
Low fat omlettes	Eggs scrambled or fried
Dry cereals	in grease
Hot cereals	
Fresh fruit	
Fresh Juices	

Once In A While
Pancakes
Waffles
French toast

(Try these with yogurt topping or fruit instead of syrup. Avoid using butter!)

SANDWICHES

Okay Selections	Selections of Concern
Sliced chicken	Hamburger
Sliced turkey	Egg salad
Skim cheeses	Reuben
Vegie/pita	Chicken salad
Lean meats	Fishburger
	Most deli meats
	Grilled hot dog
	Corn dog
	Luncheon meat
	Chicken nuggets
	Fishburger
	Patty melt

Use mustards instead of mayonnaise or butter if you need a bread spread.

BREADS AND STARCHES

Okay Selections	Selections of Concern
Bread sticks	Biscuits
Bagels	Muffins
Pretzels	French Fries
French bread	Garlic Bread
Tortillas	All chips
Pastas	Croissants/Popovers
Hard rolls	Fried Vegetables
Soft rolls	
Rice	
Wild rice	
Noodles	
Rice pilaf	
Baked potato	
Sweet potato	
Au gratin vegetables	

VEGETABLES

Okay Selections	Selections of Concern
Plain vegetables (stewed, steamed, boiled or stir fried in water or bouillon)	Buttered, Creamed, fried, sauteed or au gratin

DESSERTS

Okay Selections	Selections of Concern
Fruit compote	Ice cream
Fresh fruit	Rich desserts/pastries
Canned fruit	Custards/puddings
Sorbet	Pies/cakes
Angel food cake	
Jello desserts	
Frozen yogurt	
Sherbet	

The most important thing you can do when changing any habit is to *notice*. Eating is no different. Here's some noticing you can do in a restaurant:

Take the time to notice your true hunger level. Regardless of what you choose, eat portions that reflect your appetite.

Notice which part of the menu you look at first? Is it the salads? Low calorie special? Dessert? Do these external cues affect what you order?

Notice the messages that come into your head? Do they reflect your values or the values of your parents or other peers?

Notice whether the restaurant steers you to the bar for appetite stimulating alcohol and salty foods. If so, complain and avoid them in the future.

What are you thinking about? If it is food, is it calories? Is it about being "good" or being "bad"?

Are you influenced by the choices made by your companions?

Does cost of the dish influence what you choose?

I like "eating out" and almost everyone else I know enjoys it too. It is part of our culture–part of our socio-economic existence. It is our lifestyle. Armed with this new awareness of alternatives/choices/options you can participate fully and enjoy the joy we're entitled to experience in everything we do!

SUPERMARKET SMARTS

Do you experience a fleeting moment of confusion every time you enter a supermarket? I do. Each store has its own personality and, although layout from store to store has some consistency, each new excursion combines excitement with fear of the unknown. New products to view, ever-changing displays and seasonal decorations become elements of the psychological issues involved in how we choose to buy or not-to-buy products. No wonder we get slowed down and distracted in our search for the familiar and the new items we want or need. The typical U. S. supermarket offers more than 10,000 items to compete for your appetite and grocery dollar.

Put your anxiety on hold. Like every experience, becoming armed with some knowledge and skill can give you a more comfortable perspective during shopping excursions. They can be more successful, less painful and contribute significantly to the well being that comes with getting the most out of your food dollar.

My experience working with people making lifestyle change

has resulted in the following basic guidelines I suggest as first steps to establishing savvy shopping habits:

Whenever possible, plan your menus in advance.

Make and use a menu-coordinated shopping list.

Avoid shopping when hungry.

Shop at consumer oriented rather than sales oriented markets.

Avoid overbuying.

Beware of the supermarket enticements that draw you to the store.

Be aware of individual family preferences but don't be persuaded to sabotage your eating plan.

And now, about those lists I so casually suggested you make! Some people make lists and follow them to the letter; some people make lists and never look at them again, and some people don't need to write lists-they keep them in their head. That is human nature. If you are not a list maker or user, you might consider altering your behavior to add list making to your repertoire of lowfat lifestyle habits. Surveys show that people who shop with a list buy fewer items than those who shop without one.

Feeling helpless about list construction? I just list the products I need. My friend Mark begins by making a master sheet of food categories and duplicating it for regular use. He organizes the categories on paper with an eye to the layout of the store. Typical categories include dairy products, fruits and vegetables, meats, frozen foods, breads and cereals, staples, and non-food items.

Stick to your list to avoid impulse buying, but be flexible enough to take advantage of bargains on foods you use regularly in your lowfat lifestyle. If you find yourself tempted by foods not on your list, pause, make contact with that skinny person inside, finish the task at hand and head for the checkout line. Once you leave the store you will be reluctant to return for those "extras".

You will have more success sticking to your eating plan if you shop for groceries only once or twice a week. When possible, schedule your excursion for a time of day when you are not hungry so you will be more resistant to temptation. When you shop, buy only what you need or what you believe are bargain items important to your diet. Locate a fresh produce stand or farmer's market where you can buy fresh fruits and vegetables between major grocery outings to add a mental high akin to home gardening.

Be aware of how supermarkets are designed. Supermarket layout follows a psychological strategy that includes carefully designed traffic patterns that encourage customers to purchase those items that return a higher margin of profit to the store. Built in traps lurk at every market place. If you stick to the perimeter of the store where food items with the greatest nutrient density are usually shelved, then run down the aisles for staples, avoiding packaged foods, your chances are much better for maintaining high nutrient density with your purchases. Remember that sugary products and products with high T. V. advertising budgets are stocked at the eye level of a child and/or designed for a woman with an height of 5'4". That is why it is important to avoid taking small children to the store. For an enlightening overview of this psychology first hand, march down the cereal aisle and check out where the various products are shelved. Children (especially nagging children) will also tempt you to buy treats you don't want or need. Those high profit, empty calorie foods and toys at the checkout stand are there to encourage this nagging and impulse buying.

Plan a supermarket outing with your family, neighbors or other friends interested in a lowfat lifestyle. A group perspective can help you avoid the traps set for you by marketing experts. You can scout the place out as a team and you will all leave with a better orientation to where to find the bargains, foods that conform to dietary goals, and items that will support your improved living habits.

It has been estimated that 47 percent of all food purchases are made on impulse. The following tips can make your trip to the supermarket less impulsive, and more successful:

Think of menu planning and supermarket shopping as a hobby, not a chore.

Attach a sheet of paper with a magnet or tape to the refrigerator and keep an ongoing list of supermarket needs. Seeing a list of healthy choices in advance will strengthen your resolve on-site.

When you shop take only enough money for essentials.

Think of yourself as being on a fitness budget.

If it helps, ask a buddy who supports your change to shop with you.

Read labels carefully to check for ingredients, serving size, nutrient and calorie contents. Once you are aware of how to convert grams to calories compute empty calories of foods to determine if that purchase is really a "best buy".

Look for "whole" and "100%" grains.

Purchase low calorie, high nutrient snacks. On those rare occasions when you purchase packaged chips or cookies, choose individual servings so if you are tempted you won't eat the entire bag.

Remember that lower shelves usually offer better buys than eye level shelves.

Can or freeze fresh, in-season foods for use all year long.

When you return home ask someone else to put groceries away.

Food is an essential of life. The social, economical and psychological aspects surrounding the purchase of this life essential have a far reaching impact on the quality and longevity of your life. Invest some time and effort to make use of these and your own supermarket smarts and you will give that part of your process meaning.

LOADING THE LARDER

I find it amusing that the "old" name for a place to store foods is a "larder". It makes sense; most foods in an average kitchen are too high in fat. I also know that the high fat diet we are all now trying to avoid is a product of post-larder years. Perhaps the pre-fat day name was a promise of things to come.

Once people get some of the basic principles about how to choose between low fat and high fat foods under their mental belt I encourage them to take advantage of their commitment to use this new knowledge by going through their cupboards and refrigerator, getting rid of the grease and restocking with the foods that can make low fat food preparation an easy choice.

The following lowfat lifestyle shopping list is a place for you to start:

Meat Group Foods

Beans: canned and dry, pintos, kidney, garbanzo, navy, black
Split peas
Lentils
Refrigerated bean dip without fat added
Water pack tuna
Shrimp, scallops, lobster, crab
All fish, but especially white fish fillets
White fish steaks (to BBQ)
Lean red meat and veal
Lean pork
Boneless, skinless chicken and turkey
Ground turkey and chicken
Eggs (3 a week) and Egg Beaters
"Reduced turkey" ham, bologna, etc.
Louis Rich Turkey Breakfast Sausage (or similar product)
Tofu

Milk Group Foods

Non-fat and lowfat milk
Non-fat yogurt, plain and flavored, for cooking and eating
Lowfat yogurt for eating (if non-fat is intolerable)
Lowfat cottage cheese (Weight Watchers• is lowest)
Non-fat buttermilk
Dried buttermilk for baking
Non-fat powdered milk
Low calorie Nutrasweet cocoa mix
Evaporated skim milk (for baking and coffee)
A variety of low fat ice cream products
Weight Watchers Frozen Desserts
Dry cottage cheese (for cooking!)
Laughing Cow reduced calorie cheese
Lite Line and Weight Watchers Cheese (33-55% fat)
Farmer's, Lappi, Mozarella, String cheese from skim milk
Strongly flavored cheese for cooking (extra sharp cheddar, parmesan, etc., but cut down on amounts and mix with low fat choices)
Lean cream cheese
Light sour cream

Bread and Cereal Group Foods _____
Barley
100% stone ground whole wheat bread
Whole wheat English muffins
Whole wheat tortillas, corn tortillas-use for making chips
Whole wheat pita pocket bread
Whole wheat, pumpernickel bagels
Whole wheat pastry and bread flour (mix 1/2 with white in conventional recipes)
Frozen Belgian Waffles
Crackers: Plain RyKrisp, Norwegian thick or thin flatbread, Wasa, Melba Toast, Crackelbread, Crisp Bread, 4 Grain and other crackers that don't list oil as one of the ingredients.
Pretzels: with no oil listed
Bread sticks
Cornmeal: undegerminated, keep refrigerated
Millet
Brown rice
Wild rice
Angel food cake or mix
Bulk packaged popping corn or Weight Watchers
Corn, fresh or frozen
Pasta: whole grain, vegetable or regula-all shapes and styles
Hot cereals: Oatmeal, Wheat Hearts, Roman Meal, Oat Bran, Cream of Rye Wheatena and others labeled as whole grain, Zoom, Cream of Wheat
Cold cereals: Shredded Wheat, Grape Nut Flakes, Bran Cereals, Total Oatios, Nutri Grain, Most, whole grain puffed cereals, Granola without nuts or sweetenings, Cheerios
Rice Cakes

Fruit and Vegetable Group Foods _____
All fresh, frozen and canned vegetables (but not if packaged in oil)
All fresh, frozen and canned fruits (but not canned in syrup)
Frozen juice concentrate (for baking or sweetening)
Frozen hash browns
Salsa

Extras: _____

Butter buds
Lite salts
Diet mayonnaise
Pam
Diet sodas
Bran
Equal
Crystal Lite
Reduced calorie wines & beers
Diet margarine
Molly McButter
Bouillon/consomme
No sugar jams and syrups
Low fat soup mixes
Dry salad dressing mixes
Low or no oil salad dressings
Weight Watchers or Pritikin products (variable taste quality)
Nutrasweet and Nutrasweet flavored Gelatins and puddings.

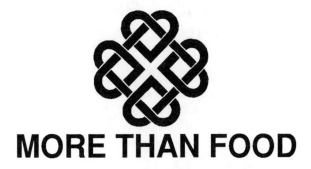

MORE THAN FOOD

The title of this book is <u>Nutrition Nuggets and More</u> and the text you have been reading about food has been permeated with reminders to exercise regularly. There is a lot of information out there to help you get started on an exercise program and you can consult the Lifestyles Resource Guide* for some of my favorites. Here, however, are some specifics on exercise related subjects that I hope will give you something to think about as you plan your workouts for the week.

* See book order form for information

TAKING A BREAK: EXERCISES TO AVOID*

You have probably noticed that along with giving people practical information about food I also encourage them to exercise regularly including occasional specifics on how, when, where and why. Here are some exercises I'd like you to *avoid*.

JUMPING on the bandwagon.
WADING through paperwork.
MAKING mountains out of molehills.
RUNNING down your friends.
BEATING around the bush.
CLIMBING the walls.
PASSING the buck.
PUSHING your luck.
SPINNING your wheels.
BEATING your head against the wall.
ADDING fuel to the fire.
DRAGGING your heels.
JUMPING to conclusions.
SIDESTEPPING your responsibilities.
FISHING for compliments.
SHIFTING the blame.
THROWING your weight around.
FOCUSING on irrelevancies.
FLYING off the handle.
CARRYING things too far.
DODGING responsibilities.
FLIRTING with disaster.

* Various sources

OPTIMUM EXERCISE LEVEL
(P.L.E.ase)

If you are in an aerobic exercise class you have probably computed your target heart rate (T. H. R.) and monitored your pulse to establish a good exercise level. That is a good thing to do once in a while but it is more important to think about exercising at a level that warms your body and increases your heart rate and respiration to levels that are comfortable but don't make you breathless. This is called your perceived level of exertion (P. L. E.).

My friend Cheryl is 40 years old so her 65-80% of maximum heart rate (220 - her age) computes to be 110 to 136 beats per minute. Once when we were jogging together and moving at a comfortable pace we both took our pulse to see how close it came to our computed target heart rate. Hers was almost 180! I thought I had a potential heart attack victim on my hands, but she was perfectly fine. We continued exercising and monitored our pulse again. Hers stayed at that high level.

Cheryl is small boned. She has small wrists and small feet and she probably has a small heart too. That smaller heart has to beat a lot more often to pump oxygenated blood to her muscles when she exercises. My friend Dave is 55 so 65-80% of his maximum computed working heart rate is 100 to 125 beats per minute. However, when we ran together and he was working at his perceived level of exertion, his heart rate barely reached minimum target levels. He's been physically active for a long time and may have a big, well developed heart that reaches a sufficient enough stroke volume per beat that it doesn't have to beat so often to get oxygen to his working muscles. I, on the other hand, find my computed target heart rate and my pulse at my perceived level of exertion are right on target with what heart rate charts say it should be. Three very different individuals, with three very different–and correct–optimum exercise levels.

Lots of factors can affect your heart rate. Exercise is part of a good health plan often prescribed by savvy physicians whose patients are on blood pressure medication and anti-depressants or other medications which can change the heart rate and make computing accurate target heart rates virtually impossible. Stress and illness can also alter heart rates.

The point is that although lots of people exercise with instructors who encourage them to keep their heart rate in their computed target range, studies have shown that using a formula to compute an effective working heart rate works for some, but obviously not all of our population.

When you exercise keep in touch with how you feel. Find that pace at which you feel so good you know you could keep moving comfortably that way for up to an hour. Fitness motivator Murray Banks encourages use of the P & P principle–puff and perspiration to monitor your workout.

Whether you choose THR, PLE or the P & P principle listen to your body. It is still the most common sense way to monitor your work and your workout–and become as fit as you can be!

(Some of the)
BENEFITS OF AEROBIC
EXERCISE

Most people who exercise regularly don't need a reason to do so. Even those who have difficulty getting started realize the most immediate benefit–feeling better about themselves. That occurs as soon as they finish their first workout and it is what keeps them going on a daily basis. My experience is that only competitive athletes are motivated by the physiological changes they can expect as they maintain their workout schedule. Everyone else likes the potential for decreased body fat, positive changes in their hunger patterns and feeling they are more in control of their life. Or as one of my clients put it, "I knew you'd encourage me to exercise and I dreaded it. Now it's the key to maintaining all my lifestyle behaviors. When I exercise regularly I want to eat sensibly and make the rest of my life manageable too.

So, even if you are not "into" the physiological and psychological benefits of aerobic exercise, I have listed some of them here so you can be aware of the internal as well as the external changes of an aerobic lifestyle. Go for it!

AEROBIC EXERCISE:

Improves	handling of excess heat
	resistance to cold

Increases	hemoglobin concentration
	density in bones
	HDL cholesterol
	glycogen storage
	stroke volume of heart
	ventricle size increases
	ventricle wall strengthens
	oxygen delivery to brain
	relieves senility
	oxygen pickup in lungs
	enzymes that burn stored body fat
	muscle mass
	burning more calories at rest
	making it easier to exercise
	aerobic threshold
	higher exercise levels
	more calories burned
	more use of fat calories
	ability to handle stress (endorphins)

Decreases	blood triglycerides
	blood pressure
	resting heart rate
	body fat
	stress (attitude)
	load on the heart
	muscle use of stored glycogen
	hypoglycemia

It Also provides an emotional lift that will have you coming back for more!

BICYCLING FOR FITNESS

So much interest and information has been available about aerobics in recent years that I make the mistake of assuming everyone knows the kinds of activities that will give you aerobic fitness. So, when I was asked during a recent lecture, "Is biking a good way to get fit?", I was surprised.

I remember the challenge of my first bike and the sense of pride I had when I was finally able to balance it the full length of the straightaway on the street where I grew up. Later it provided instant mobility to school, the home of a friend, or transportation and escape to a secret hideaway. Biking ranks right up there as one of the top three childhood activities I have been able to carry over into my adult fitness routine. I am not alone. It is now the second most popular recreational fitness activity after swimming.

These days there are as many bike styles, shapes, colors, speeds and prices as there are prospective buyers. If you have decided to take up biking for fitness there are a few things to consider before you make your decision about what kind of bike to buy. The first is the terrain where you will be cycling and the way you will be incorporating your cycling into your lifestyle.

If recreational cycling is your goal, a one- or three-speed bike may serve your needs–if you bike on a flat surface. If you want to tour, commute, or if hills are a part of your route a ten speed bike will be more suitable. All-terrain or mountain bikes, with their fat tires, straight handlebars, and substantial frame are good all around choices for city streets, country roads, commuting, exercising or going off road. Regardless of which one you choose it is essential that your gears operate smoothly, especially when you ride in hilly terrain.

There are two kinds of handlebars available. Upright handlebars allow you to sit up straight and see better; they are more practical for recreational riding. Dropped handlebars are more suitable for touring or commuting because lowering your body decreases wind resistance and gives you a more stable riding position.

Once you have your bike, seat placement will be the most critical factor in determining your cycling comfort. When you are on the bike seat (known as the saddle) your knee should be slightly bent when your foot is at the bottom of the pedaling revolution. Any other seat position sacrifices leg power. You will find a variety of saddles available and that your choice becomes one of trial and error, although the more comfortable seats usually cost more.

Aerobic riding technique means pedalling steadily or "spinning" the wheels fast enough so your large lower muscles are always moving, but not so fast you can't keep up with the spin. A gear that allows you to maintain your training heart rate while spinning at 70-90 revolutions per minute will assure an optimum aerobic workout. If you can carry on a conversation while exercising and don't become breathless, you are exercising at what is described as a "perceived level of exertion."

For safety, wear a comfortable helmet, and gloves that give you a good grip on the handlebars. Lights and reflectors are essential for night riding. By law, a bike is a vehicle, so a knowledge of traffic laws is mandatory. You must ride on the right side of the street, signalling all turns, slowing and stopping with your left hand. For safety, unless you have a mountain bike, avoid potholes and gutters. Regardless of what kind of bike you use when you are on the street you will need to watch for car doors opening along the side of the road, and buses that may be pulling in to the curb.

Know how to make simple adjustments, change a flat tire, and keep your bike tuned. Tire pressure should be checked once a week because under- or over-inflated tires cause flats. If you don't feel comfortable doing your own maintenance be sure to have your bike checked regularly by a good mechanic. My brother Buzz owns a bike store in Colorado and he regularly sponsors bicycling workshops and clinics that teach these skills. The one I attended proved these events are a great place to pick up tips and meet other people who share your love for the outdoors. Like most quality stores, Buzz also hosts a riding club and provides a variety of route maps for touring in the area.

If time for yourself is a premium or you live in a climate where it is difficult to bicycle year round or you are just not an outdoors person, a stationary bicycle may be a more appropriate choice for biking for fitness. The guidelines for choosing a stationary bike focus more on durability, smooth and quiet operation, and maintenance requirements. All these bikes have upright handlebars and adjustable seats so they can be used by all members of the family. They vary in price from $50 to $2500 and the price usually reflects the accouterments. About $200-$400 is an adequate investment for the home user who wants to exercise for about 30-40 minutes a day. Choose a bike that has a large, balanced flywheel (the spinning wheel on the front of the bike) and a durable and efficient braking system (that part of the bike that provides the friction to control the speed of the flywheel. Be sure to try several models before you make a purchase and choose the one you feel most comfortable climbing onto several times in a row.

Regardless of what kind of bike you choose your workout should include a warmup and cooldown. Biking brings all the muscle groups of the legs into play, so stretching your hamstrings and calves before and after your ride will relax your muscles, help prevent injury and ease any aches and pains. To prevent post-ride aches and pains begin and finish with several minutes of easy pedalling.

If you have chosen to do your bicycling outside you may be interested in cycling clubs that offer a variety of activities for bikers of all ages. They advertise their activities in local bike shops. Even if you choose not to get deeply involved in this fine activity you will soon learn there is nothing quite as exhilarating as riding down a country road with the wind in your face, or a leisurely trek through the neighborhood in the company of friends or family, or the power of physically transporting yourself as you move from place to place in the course of your daily activities. For me, biking has become more than a way to travel between two points and to exercise. It gave me the opportunity to experience the world at close range, to become a part of the landscape.

My recreational cycling takes me on day long trips with a pack on my bike filled with lots of energy producing foods. They include a filled water bottle to replenish fluids lost by sweat and respiration and light weight, high carbohydrate, easy-to-pack snacks. I stop at roadside stands for other foods and make every rest stop into a picnic.

Try your own bike excursion soon. You can recapture memories of childhood too.

ROPE SKIPPING
FOR HEALTH

Lois was a rope-skipping champion. I had never seen an adult move like she did. She could make a simple rope revolution seem like magic as she went through complicated dance-like patterns that challenged her coordination as well as her fitness. When she could get two people to power a pair of ropes for her, the movements became almost mystical as she danced in and out of their way with a finesse that left my mouth gaping!

Lois was really fit and was testimony that rope skipping is as effective a fitness exercise as you can find. She talked as she skipped and reminded me that in addition to being convenient and inexpensive it is an exercise that produces the greatest fitness in the shortest amount of time. In fact, one study she cited showed 10 minutes of rope-skipping to be as effective as a 30-minute jogging program.

Rope skipping follows all the rules of aerobics. It uses your major muscle groups and quickly increases your respiration to a perceived level of exertion. When practiced 20 minutes a day five days a week it can increase cardiovascular efficiency (VO2 max) 23-31%. In addition it enhances coordination and balance, two components of a balanced exercise program very often overlooked.

The downside is that it is not for everybody. Jumping rope puts extra stress on the knees and hip joints. And because it is an impact activity it may be limited as a fitness regimen, especially on less than optimum floor surfaces, to people who are at optimum weights and have healthy lower bodies.

If you want to try it, you will need a rope long enough to reach from armpit to armpit while passing under the feet. Sash cord from hardware stores is suitable if it holds its shape while being twirled. Properly sized ready-made jump ropes are most suitable and there is a wide variety available at most fitness stores.

My resources produced this progressive program recommended by Physiologist, Kaare Rodahl :

First Week: Warm up by jumping in place (on both feet together) 50 to 100 times without the rope. Next, skip the rope 50 times, at whatever speed you like. (Beginners will find it easier at first to lift both feet off the ground at the same time.) On the first day that is plenty! On the second, third, fourth and fifth days add ten skips per day. By week's end (a five day week is ample) you will be doing 90 skips without stopping.

Second Week: Warm up without the rope by doing 50 slow hops. But note: This week, abandon that feet-together hop and step over the flying rope one foot at a time, left-right, left-right as if jogging in place. Start with 100 such skips. Each day add ten more. Final day, 140.

Third Week: Warm up as usual. Skip 100 times without stopping. Rest 15 to 30 seconds. Skip another 200 times.

Fourth Week and on: By now, improved endurance should enable you to skip with less effort. The object now is to skip fast enough or long enough to get a bit out of breath, the result of making the heart call for more oxygen.

Ultimate Goal: Skip and rest, skip and rest, until the day you can do 500 consecutive skips in five minutes.

Do's and Don'ts: When you skip, relax. Look straight ahead. Jump just high enough–about an inch–for the rope to pass under your feet. Wear sneakers or similar shoes, no heels. Some of the new aerobic shoes with a cushioned bottom are perfect. Land on the balls of your feet. Don't use much arm movement, the hands should describe a circle about eight to ten inches in diameter. Skip on a thick carpet or lawn, never on a hard surface. Be sure to warm up the legs before and after your workout by circling the feet, pointing and flexing at the ankles (this protects the forefront of the shin) and stretch out the calves by standing in a position that protects the back but hyperextends the muscles in the calves.

If you are like my daughter your enthusiasm for this new sport will take your body beyond the limits it can endure in the early days of a new activity. Becca discovered it was fun to skip with the ropes I purchased for my studio. Although I cautioned her, she kept at it for 30 minutes claiming she had done a good warmup, was wearing proper shoes and was on a sprung floor. The next day she could hardly walk. I don't need to tell you that her enthusiasm died as quickly as it was born. So, be sure to follow the recommended progression no matter how fit you are. Then, perhaps you will be like me and carry a rope in your suitcase for those days when you are on the road but can't get out on the road. Like Lois we can be fleet footed too.

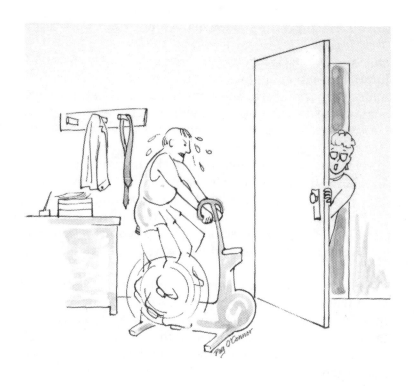

"Only 106 calories until your power lunch, Mr. Bailey."

CROSS TRAINING

Whenever I lecture about beginning a regular exercise program people in the audience ask me if there is one exercise they should choose over another. I don't think there is. In fact I encourage people to cross train for a balanced lifestyle. Cross training means exercising in more than one way. Taking aerobic dance at 9:00 every morning is not a balanced and varied way to work out no matter how much you love it. So when you look at other possibilities for supplementing your current program or when you wonder where to begin, I suggest you look at the activities you enjoyed as a child.

Swimming, bicycling, roller and/or ice skating, rowing, skiing, (especially cross country skiing) hiking, walking and jogging continue to be the most popular aerobic sports with which people choose to cross train. I have a rowing machine and a bicycle at my home, so on days when the weather is inclement I put on a record and dance away in my living room, then jump on the bike for a couple of songs and do the same with my rowing machine. Before I know it I have 40 minutes of aerobic exercise under my belt.

I recently tried one of the new stair climbing machines at the local health club. Talk about a workout! I have a cousin on the East Coast who has also taken to stair climbing; we enjoy the friendly competition of counting and comparing the number of floors we have climbed each month. I have also discovered that I maintain contact with a wider assortment of friends by changing my workout regularly. I bike with Bill and Lea, jog with Cheryl, Beebe and Diane, swim with my daughter and dance with the friends in my aerobic dance class.

Aside from the obvious benefits of exercising a variety of major muscle groups when you vary your exercise patterns, it is a great way to prevent the injuries that can occur when muscles are overworked. And, speaking of injuries, I had one myself recently when I jumped off a low wall in the dark and landed on a rock, twisting my ankle somewhat seriously. After resting my ankle for a few days I was especially happy that I was already well acquainted with several options for exercising. I was able to maintain my aerobic fitness while I nursed my ankle to health by focusing more on my swimming, stationary cycling and stair climbing and less on jogging and dancing.

Tap into your own memories and resources for exercise. Remember, it is easiest to maintain your commitment when you plan in advance. And, by working out in many different ways, you can describe yourself as an all around athlete. I do.

STRETCH FOR RUNNING

I occasionally conduct stretch clinics to help runners increase their flexibility in preparation for the summer season of weekend races. After each one of these events people ask me if I would put on paper the routine I suggested they use before and/or after their workout. It has always been difficult for me to put motion into words but here is what I came up with. (Note: You don't have to be a runner to get a lot out of these stretches!)

STANDING STRETCHES
TO OPEN YOUR CHEST AND LUNGS
Standing with feet shoulder-width apart...
Inhale deeply while raising the arms overhead to allow for fuller expansion of the lungs. Exhale and let the arms drop to your sides. Repeat the inhalation then lace the fingers above the head with the hands turned palms to ceiling. Bend the right knee and gently lean to the left, keeping the elbows outside the ears. Exhale. As you inhale again, straighten to vertical and as you exhale bend the left knee, and lean to the right. Inhale as you come to vertical, and as you exhale drop your arms to the starting position.

TO RELAX AND LOOSEN UP
Standing with feet shoulder-width apart...
Drop your chin to your chest, slump your shoulders, drop your chest forward, relax your knees and slowly roll down until you are "hanging" from your hips with your arms loose and forward. Be sure to keep your weight forward on the balls of your feet and your knees relaxed, not "locked".

Take a deep breath. As you exhale, relax deeper and feel this stretch in the hamstrings and lower back. Repeat with another deep breath. Roll up slowly straightening the spine "one vertebrae at a time" until you are fully erect.

LEFT AND RIGHT HAMSTRING STRETCH
Place the left foot over the right using the left toe to balance yourself and keeping the left heel off the floor to keep the hips aligned. Repeat the "dropover" process described above. Roll up slowly.

Repeat the movement with the right foot over the left.

If you have difficulty keeping your balance, do this with your hand on a chair or wall.

TO OPEN CHEST AND SHOULDER BLADE AREA
Lace the fingers behind the back, and with the knees slightly bent and while inhaling, lift the hands behind the back to stretch the muscles across the chest and between the shoulders.

As you exhale, bend the right knee and twist gently to the right. Inhale again as you return to center. Bend the left knee and repeat the process with a gentle twist to the left.

Release the hands and shake them out.

TO STRETCH QUADRICEPS AND HIP FLEXORS
Standing on your right foot, balance yourself by holding onto something with your left hand. Bend your left knee so

your foot elevates behind you and grab it with your right hand. Inhale deeply. As you exhale, push your left hip slightly forward as you push your foot against your hand. Do not overstretch. Release the foot and repeat on the other side.

Note: Many people do this stretch with the right hand to right foot and left hand to left foot. I prefer my method because it allows the hip joint to more correctly rotate outward.

FLOOR STRETCHES
TO OPEN THE GROIN AREA
Sit with the soles of your feet together, but with your back straight so you don't sit in a slumped position. While holding your feet with your hands (but not pulling on your toes, which would "sickle" your feet in an unnatural position), inhale deeply. Put your elbows on your legs above or below the knees and as you exhale fully, gently push down with your elbows. Repeat for several deep breaths.

TO STRETCH THE BACK MUSCLES
Sitting with the soles of the feet together, slide the feet away from your body until the feet begin to separate at the heels. This position frees the hip area and increases the stretch.

For the upper back and neck...
Drop the chin to the chest. (If you have never stretched like this before this movement may create a tingling sensation in the back of your neck.) Inhale deeply. As you exhale, see if you can drop the head forward a little more. If this movement is comfortable, put your hands on the crown of your head to add a little extra weight to the stretch. Be sure you don't hunch your shoulders. Repeat the deep breath progressions trying to ease and relax tension normally held in the neck and shoulder areas.

For the lower back...
Slide your hands under your heels to elevate them slightly and to provide leverage to pull the body forward toward the

feet. Think of extending your head past your heels. Repeat the breath progressions trying to move a little farther forward each time you exhale.

TO STRETCH SIDES OF BACK, HAMSTRINGS AND GROIN AREA

Sitting in a front hurdle position (one leg out to the side and the other folded in front of you),* inhale, and as you exhale, gently twist your body in the direction of the bent knee. Repeat.

Inhale and as you exhale bend sideways over your long leg for a stretch to the side of the body. Repeat deep breathing routine to relax into the stretch.

Turn so you are facing the extended leg. Inhale, and as you exhale gently lean out and over the leg.

Repeat the progression on the other side.

Caution: A hurdle position with the bent leg behind can be very hard on your knees and should be approached with caution.

KNEELING STRETCHES

TO STRETCH THE CALVES, ACHILLES AREA AND HAMSTRINGS

Assume a position known as "all fours." Press up into an inverted "V" with the weight evenly distributed on your hands and feet. While bending your right knee, gently push the heel of your left foot into the floor. Think about alternating lifting your tail bone to the ceiling and tucking it under.

Repeat the stretch on the other side.

*For people uncomfortable on all fours these exercises can be done by leaning the forearms against a wall with the toes placed about 18 inches from the wall.

TO EXTEND THE STRETCH LOWER IN THE LEG

Keep one heel on the floor, then bend that leg slightly. The amount of bending the knee can take is dependent on the angle of the body and the amount of stretch the muscles can sustain, so be gentle.

Repeat the movement on the other side.

Bring the feet together using a toe-heel-toe-heel movement. Bend the knees slightly and roll up slowly as you inhale. Exhale after you come to a full standing position. When you are standing, inhale deeply as you lift your arms overhead, as you did in the first exercise.

You have now come full circle and will be very relaxed. If you are starting a run, sigh deeply and start off slowly. If you have finished your workout, walk around slowly and enjoy the beauty that surrounds you.

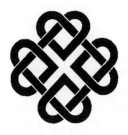

MISCELLANEOUS
MUSINGS

Nutrition Nuggets became More than a vision when I began reviewing the articles about exercise and nutrition I had written for various publications the past five years and saw there was some continuity to the material. In addition to writing about "major" nutrition issues like dieting and fat and sugar and fiber and label reading, I discovered I had occasionally focused on specifics. Miscellaneous Musings is a small collection of the most popular of these mini-subjects. Muse and enjoy!

DAD'S WISDOM

The following was found among my father's papers after he passed away. I don't know the source. Dad was a physician who specialized in chest medicine and he was an advocate of returning his heart attack patients to an active lifestyle. Sadly he knew little about the role of diet in heart disease (except to insist his patients maintain a "normal" weight). He loved and ate high fat foods and succumbed to heart disease himself at the age of 72.

1. Go less, sleep more.
2. Ride less, walk more.
3. Talk less, think more.
4. Scold less, praise more.
5. Waste less, give more.
6. Eat less, chew more.
7. Clothe less, bathe more.
8. Idle less, play more.
9. Worry less, laugh more.
10. Preach less, practice more.

MARTY'S SHINSPLINTS

When I returned to teaching my aerobic dance exercise class after a lengthy absence to fulfill some lecture commitments, I noticed Marty wasn't moving with the same enthusiasm and energy as she had in the past. Marty was an avid aerobic dance student. In fact, she had told me several weeks earlier that on the days I didn't teach she went to a class in a church a couple of blocks away so she could workout at least once a day. I had cautioned my students about doing the same kind of exercise too often–I am an advocate of cross training–but there was no convincing Marty. She only liked to dance and having lost the twelve pounds she had once gained when she had to stop working out for three months she was determined never to gain weight again.

After class I asked her if she was okay. She hesitated then confessed, "Well, I've been having some soreness in my legs, and quite frankly they start hurting about ten minutes into the workout. They *kill* me when I go down stairs but usually feel better in the morning." I asked her to point to the area of soreness. As I expected, she pointed to her shins. Marty had what are known as shinsplints, the bane of any exercise program. Shinsplints are particularly an issue for students and instructors of aerobic dance.

Shinsplints, a term used to describe a number of syndromes that affect the lower leg, are usually described as a nagging ache in the muscles that surround the shin bone-sharp enough to hurt, but dull enough to be able to continue an exercise program. The soreness Marty was feeling was probably from swollen muscles pulling away from the shin bone. The pain left her overnight, but resuming her exercise program brought it right back. Mild shinsplint pain usually isn't serious enough to cause alarm, but if not taken seriously, it can develop into something worse, including stress fractures of the lower leg.

Shinsplints are one of the most common running maladies and one of the most frequently reported aerobic-dance injuries. Shinsplints are usually caused by exercising on hard surfaces, improper or ill fitting footwear, poor technique and failure to warm both the front and back of the lower leg sufficiently before a workout. Since my classes are held on a "sprung" floor which is considered the most ideal surface, I asked Marty if she had new shoes. She did, but they were the same model she had been wearing in the past and she was pretty comfortable with them. I asked her if she was still going to class elsewhere. She was. I asked her about the surface there. She said her other class was on a cement floor–the worst surface for a dance exercise class, especially if the class includes any jumping movement.

It was too late for Marty to do what is necessary to help prevent shinsplints. The best prevention of shinsplints is in the preparation, the warmup for your aerobic activity. It includes wearing the appropriate shoes for less than optimum surfaces, warming up the lower leg by pointing and flexing the ankle, tapping the toe and doing foot rotations, gently stretching the calve muscles by leaning forward against a wall with the heels in contact with the floor or by going to "all fours" (not on your hands and knees but on your hands and feet) and alternately pressing the heels to the floor.

Rest is the best cure for shin splints, but it is the hardest treatment for avid students to endure. I encouraged Marty to avoid dance exercise for awhile. I knew her husband worked out on an exercise bike and rowing machine at home, and suggested she maintain her fitness by using the machines on alternate days, icing her shins before and after each workout. I also suggested she take aspirin–two of them 3 times a day–to reduce any inflammation and swelling. As her legs improved applications of ten minutes of wet heat followed by twenty minutes of ice would help. I stressed the importance of checking with a physican if she didn't have some relief within a few days to see if she had a stress fracture or tendonitis. I encouraged her to treat her legs more gently now to avoid a more serious injury and more lengthy medical treatment later.

Marty stopped coming to my class, but she continued with the other class until her legs hurt so badly she could hardly walk. She paid her dues with a lengthy layoff from both classes. Happily, in time her legs healed and when she returned to class she was equipped with smash-before-use ice packs which she used before and after class, and a pair of leg warmers to assure her muscles stayed warm and flexible while she worked out. The best part of her "recovery" was the transition she made to cross training. She discovered that the bike and rowing machines were a viable alternative to her dance exercise class, and she worked up a routine where she switched from one to another throughout a 40 minute period so she didn't get bored.

Not everyone who gets shinsplints is as lucky as Marty was. New shoes and a poor workout surface notwithstanding, the significant predisposing factor in her injury was her desire to exercise more than she needed to for fitness' sake. Health professionals are now saying that when we run more than three miles a day or exercise more than five hours a week we are doing it for reasons other than mental or physical fitness. Overexercising is overstressing the body, and if it doesn't show up as physical discomfort or pain it often leads to emotional illness. After more than a dozen years in the dance exercise field the issue that concerns me most is the belief that more is better. In an effort to exercise for weight management–to balance extra calories in by overexercising later to burn them off–we are predisposing ourselves to eating disorders by participating in a subtle binge-purge process. Shinsplints are giving way to back pain and loss of the lean mass that burns calories. Emotionally we are tied into believing that if we get our bodies small enough everything else in our lives will fall into place. So exercise becomes the quick fix for a variety of emotional issues.

Take care of yourself. Remember that discomfort and pain are signals that something is wrong. We have a projected lifespan that goes into our eighties. Let's all be moving when we get there!

ABOUT BREAKFAST

I've heard "breakfast is the most important meal of the day" as long as I can remember, yet for most people I meet breakfast gets no respect. "Haven't got time", "breakfast is boring", or "I'm not hungry in the morning", are the most frequent excuses I hear for ignoring this important meal. Then I hear complaints about weight gain from these same folks–folks who admit they often pacify the hunger that attacks later in the morning with donuts or other traditional mid-morning snacks that are usually high in fat, cholesterol and calories. They talk about their self defeating behaviors and wonder why they can't avoid poor eating patterns.

Whoever advised you to eat breakfast probably didn't know a thing about biochemistry–but it was sound advice. When you begin your day without breakfast you are asking your body to run on nutrients and calories you ate at least 12 hours earlier. You wouldn't start a long trip with your bag half packed or your gas tank on empty, so why start your day that way?

I have clients who avoid breakfast because it gets them started on an eating binge that continues throughout the day. It makes sense. Breakfasts loaded with refined sugars and caffeine are the ones that trigger an insulin response that often leaves you craving more to eat. They feel unable to regulate their food intake once they start eating. Most of these same people admit that it is no longer the case when they get in the habit of eating a balanced low fat, low sugar, high fiber meal that includes a small amount of protein. That is the kind of breakfast that can give you a good start on necessary nutrients and maintain glucose levels that help prevent mood swings.

Some recent studies show that we burn breakfast calories more efficiently than those provided by any other meal because our metabolic rate (calorie burning capacity) is higher in the morning than the rest of the day. Other studies show that a light breakfast (a piece of whole grain toast and juice) before an early a.m. workout will pump your body with extra fat burning energy. Still other studies show that eating oat bran in the morning can decrease "bad" LDL cholesterol levels–if the remainder of the diet follows the guidelines for reduced fat. That is a good reason to return to picking up that famous round cereal box that has remained a best seller through the years despite the onslaught of sugar cereals.

After my early morning workout I shower, then have a meal of whole grain cereal, low fat milk or yogurt and fresh fruit to get me off to the kind of start that assures I am at my best levels of mental and physical health. Whether you work out early in the morning or not, this same breakfast can give you one serving from each of the milk, grain and fruits and vegetable groups to stoke you with nutrients and fiber without an expenditure of many calories.

Breaking Breakfast Traditions
Breakfast does not have to be "traditional." I know lots of people who like dinner leftovers at breakfast for a filling

meal that is neither boring nor too much trouble. In the Gates kitchen some popular leftover breakfasts include pizza, soup and toast, pasta, rice dishes and lowfat fruit pies.

For an easy to prepare healthy breakfast stock your kitchen with frozen Belgian waffles, whole wheat bagels and English muffins, a variety of whole grain breads, non-sugary cereals (especially oatmeal), and a variety of whole grain flours for cooking pancakes and other breakfast treats. If you have a non stick waffle iron or electric skillet it is easy to prepare a low fat meal.

Don't ignore breakfast. A little creativity and ingenuity first thing in the morning can give you an initial boost of energy and mood elevating satisfaction to improve your performance throughout your day.

Here are some of the more popular breakfast suggestions I've shared with my students:

Morning Pizza
Spread Lavosh or other crackers with low in fat cottage cheese and sliced fruit. Heat it in the microwave or broil it in your toaster oven.

Low Fat Blintzes
Put a dollop of low fat cottage cheese that has been mixed with a non-sweetened jam or conserve in the middle of a whole wheat tortilla. Roll, then heat it in the microwave. You can put the same ingredients in pocket bread for a different texture.

Waffles are a favorite in my house for the base of an elegant and delicious low fat breakfast. I can prepare a 14% fat waffle using a packaged multi-grain mix cooked on a teflon coated grill. I make a large batch of these and freeze the extras. In an emergency I've purchased frozen belgian waffles which are about 28% fat–still an excellent choice when smothered with low fat toppings. I've tried all kinds of toppings, but my

favorites are:
- fruit (fresh, frozen or canned in its own juice)
- non-fat yogurt mixed with low fat cream cheese
- non-fat yogurt mixed with low fat ricotta cheese
- ricotta cheese mixed with low sugar jellies
- low sugar jellies sweetened with fruit juice

EGGS FOR BREAKFAST
As I've moved to a lowfat lifestyle I eat less than the recommended three eggs a week, but when I do have a craving for them I cook them the non-fat way by poaching them or cooking them in a teflon coated skillet. If I scramble eggs I decrease the yolks and add a couple extra egg whites to the batter to fluff them up and increase the volume. Sometimes I make the dish even lower in fat by stir frying fresh vegetables in boullion or water before adding the eggs.

HOME MADE GRANOLA
Most packaged or bulk granolas are high in fat and sugar. You can make your own healthier version by combining
Oats
Raisins
Low fat, non sugar cereal,
Low fat powdered milk
A FEW carob or chocolate drops

When I encounter someone who tells me he or she doesn't have time for breakfast but is willing to drink a breakfast on the run, I suggest some of the following mixtures:

FRUIT SLUSH
Combine 1/2 cup fresh fruit, 1/2 cup skim milk, 1/2 cup crushed ice, dash of honey or package of Equal, and vanilla or almond extract.

Combine ingredients in a blender and process at highest speed for about a minute.

FROZEN YOGURT SHAKE
Chop, then freeze a banana. In a blender mix the frozen banana, 1/2 cup non-fat vanilla or other flavored yogurt, 2 tablespoons un-reconstituted frozen apple juice or passion fruit juice and 1/2 cup crushed ice. Modify this recipe by omitting the frozen juice and adding an envelope of sugar free cocoa.

FROM THE STORE
Instant oatmeal and instant Cream of Wheat
Toaster Pastry
Corn flakes, Oatios and other low in sugar cereals

OTHER BREAKFASTS ON THE RUN
Apples
Hard boiled eggs
Saltines and peanut butter (spread very thinly)
Home made Granola
V-8 juice and whole wheat toast
Low fat whole wheat bran muffins
Corn Tortillas that have been dried in a microwave or oven, then covered with low fat cheese and heated until the cheese melts.

BEYOND CHARCOAL COOKING

Whether you are a lover of the outdoors or not, nothing is more tempting to the senses than food cooked on an outdoor grill. The fragrance of the open fire, the sound of sizzling foods and sight of picnic-inspired recipes often trigger memories of past pleasurable taste sensations and events in and out of party settings.

I was recently wary of accepting a late hour invitation to grill some fresh fish on the barbecue of some friends. I was so hungry the thought of waiting for the coals to heat up and the food to cook triggered my impatience. Imagine my surprise when the food appeared ten minutes after my arrival. It was cooked to perfection on a controlled-heat gas grill. It tasted wonderful.

If you want to experiment with a cooking technique that goes beyond the time-tested charcoal, create some sensational tastes by burning hard wood or aromatic wood chips and vines with your charcoal or gas coals. The wood chips don't replace the charcoal, but, used sparingly, can create special flavors. You will need to soak the chips in water before placing them on the hot coals. For a milder flavor put dry chips directly on the coals and replenish them as needed.

Gourmet food shops and mail order catalogs sell these trendy flavor enhancers. They are expensive, but worthy of special events. Some of the more familiar ones include:

Aromatic wood or flavor	Use for
Mesquite	Duck or lamb
Hickory (southern cooking)	Ham, pork, beef
Alderwood (Pacific NW)	Seafood, especially salmon
Fruitwoods	Poultry, game
Grapevine	Poultry, seafood,
Rosemary	All fish
Seaweed	Anything
Apple	

And, having given you these hints about gourmet grilling, remember the key to non-gas grilling success is timing–knowing when the coals are ready and how long to cook the food.

Before you start, coat your grilling rack with non-stick spray then set it about 6 inches above the coals. The coals should be packed closely together in a diameter a little larger than the food you will be cooking. It will take about 30 minutes for the coals to become hot enough to cook your food.

Lower-in-fat hot dogs or meat can be cooked on the grill right over the pile of coals. If you are cooking thinner cuts of meats or fish, spread your coals over a wider area so the food won't burn before it is cooked.

I enjoy pre-cooking vegetables in the microwave then putting them on the grill for a few minutes before serving to add the outdoor flavor that makes all foods taste wonderful. I serve on bright paper plates and use a variety of napkins. Whether two or twenty, fair weather or foul, outdoor cooking is party time. May you enjoy your own soon.

WRAPPING
UP BREAD

While your choice of bread may not be a high priority when you choose foods in keeping with a lowfat lifestyle it is an important part of the U. S. Dietary Goal that encourages a diet that is higher in fiber. You already know some of the benefits of adding this "staff of life" to your diet. The myth that bread contributes to an overfat body has been overturned. But bread contributes more than fiber to our diet.

In addition to fiber the bread (and cereal) group of foods also provide us with important B vitamins, and trace minerals. For example, bread contains the trace mineral copper, the catalyst necessary to incorporate the iron essential for the production of red blood cells. About 80% of the copper in whole wheat is found in the chaff which is discarded in most commercial bread *manufacturing*. About 33% of the thiamin (Vitamin B 1), 42% of the riboflavin (Vitamin B 2), 50% of the pantothenic acid (Vitamin B 5), 73% of the pyridoxine (Vitamin B6), and 86% of the niacin (Vitamin B 3) are in the chaff and the germ or bottom of the whole wheat and are also discarded when whole wheat kernel bread is "refined".

Most people think they are buying unrefined whole wheat when they buy whole wheat bread. They are not. If you were to go out into a wheat field and shake the kernels off the top of the wheat into a basket, the contents of the basket would be whole wheat in its purest form. If you then crumbled or mashed it a little, then blew on it, the chaff (or husk) would blow right off the kernels. Since up to 15% of the wheat kernels is removed by this simple process, even stone ground whole wheat bread, the purest form available in your supermarket, is refined to some degree. If the remaining part of the wheat kernel is ground and refined to the point where 20% is removed, even more of these important vitamins and minerals disappear.

By law, wheat can be refined up to 10% and still be described as "whole wheat". When you buy a typical loaf of 100% whole wheat bread you are probably getting only about 40% to 50% of the original minerals that were in the grain before the refining process began.

How much better is 40% or 50% than 20%? Not much, really. But the difference is significant enough that most bakers enrich bread that has been refined more than 20%. When they do, they are required to add only thiamin, riboflavin, niacin and iron. They do not have to replace the copper and other trace minerals or the other B vitamins.

When you buy bread, read the label. If the first ingredient is not 100% stone ground whole wheat, you are not getting a true whole wheat bread no matter what it is called.

Also be aware that many "whole wheat breads" contain five or six different flours. Even though stone ground whole wheat may be the first ingredient it may be only 20% of the bread or bread product. The remaining ingredients may be enriched (refined) flour (white flour), rye flour, soy flour and this flour and that flour. There is an advantage to a mixed flour bread; the combined grains do provide a more complete protein than in a whole wheat bread. Although this is often a selling point emphasized by bread marketeers, it is not the reason health educators encourage it to be an important part of your diet.

For many years dieters avoided bread like the plague, thinking bread was a key factor in promoting obesity. We've since learned that fat is the culprit that contributes to weight. A 100% stone ground whole wheat bread has a satisfying taste that provides bulk without calories and should be a part of every meal. That about wraps up bread.

ABOUT ENRICHED
AND
FORTIFIED FOODS

More and more foods, including bread, are being attractively packaged with labels that extol their virtues because they are "enriched" or "fortified." I was walking Cal through a supermarket excursion. Since he was interested in selecting the most nourishing foods for his dollar he asked if these words meant these foods are good buys. This is what I told him.

When grains are refined and processed–to make bread, corn meal, flour or cereal, for example–the grain is essentially "beat up." This causes a loss of certain nutrients. "Enriched" is the term used to describe the addition of some of the nutrients lost during the process. In some products these nutrients are only partially replaced, but in whole grains more nutrients are added than the grain started with. The nutrients usually added to these products include thiamin, niacin, riboflavin and iron. They are added in amounts set by government standards. I call enriched bread products "air breads." A dietitian friend, Candy Cummings, tells her audiences that Wonder Bread got its name when they beat the grains up, losing nutrients along the way, then added others back in, looked at the product and said, "I wonder if this is still bread!"

Enriched white flour, pasta and rice are good choices nutrient-wise and they are almost always low in fat. They are lower on my preferred list than whole grain products because of their decreased fiber content.

"Fortified" is the word used to describe foods in which nutrients are added that were not there before the foods were processed. Most cereals are fortified with lots of vitamins and minerals, especially iron. These do increase the nutritional value of the food. Milk is usually fortified with Vitamin D, the vitamin we get from being in the sunshine. The added Vitamin D enhances the absorption of the calcium in milk, especially for those growing children and adults who don't spend a lot of time outdoors.

I told Cal I believe use of these terms on labels is deceptive. Adding a lot of vitamins and minerals to a food does not mean that it is more healthy for you. You still have to check the label for the fat and sugar content. Many fortified cereals on the market are high in sugar, but if they were stacked up against other cereals that are higher in fiber and not so fortified, the "junk food" cereals would appear to be better choices. In fact, a Consumer Reports study on breads showed "air breads" to be more in depth nutritionally than whole grain products that didn't have a lot of honey and sugar but did have a lot of fiber. That is a good example of how information can be used to tell you something that seems important, but in the total picture is somewhat irrelevant.

The Center for Science in the Public Interest is always on the lookout for the misuse of these terms. That is why I encourage membership (it includes their informative newsletter) in this highly regarded consumer organization. (Write to CSPI, 1501 Sixteenth St. NW, Washington, DC 20036).

Remember, there is no magic in foods. There is nothing

intrinsically wrong with fortified and enriched products. The use of these terms to create misleading advertising is wrong. Again, it is back to basics: Fresh fruits and vegetables, whole grains–foods prepared and served in as close as possible to their original form.

And, as I told Cal, read and understand what labels tell you, but don't buy by the way labels sell you.

THE PRIZE WINNER
IS CANOLA OIL!

While looking over the vast array of gleaming golden oils on the shelves of the supermarket a friend of mine came upon an oil she'd never heard of before–canola oil. "Where does it come from?", she asked me, "The canola tree?" "What is it and why did my grocer tell me it was a better choice for food preparation?"

Canola oil was formulated in 1980. It is a hybrid variety of rapeseed oil, used for years in Europe and approved in 1985 by the FDA for the U. S. market. It was introduced to the American market by Procter & Gamble when they reformulated Puritan, one of their company brands of vegetable oil.

Canola oil is lower in saturated fat than other common vegetable oils, is highly monounsaturated and also has a substantial amount of the omega-3 fatty acids found in fish oils. With its delicate taste and versatility, you will be seeing more canola oil turning up on supermarket shelves.

Procter & Gamble's advertising for Puritan says it has 50%

less saturated fat than other leading oils.They can make that claim because canola oil contains only 6% saturated fat versus 13% for corn oil and 15% for soybean oil. Since most data indicate that decreasing total fat in the diet, particularly saturated fat, is vital in preventing heart disease, canola oil is a wise choice in recipes that require fat.

More important, however, is the fact that canola oil is also high in monounsaturated fat. Diet research has shown that people who include monounsaturates in their diets can lower the levels of LDL (bad) cholesterol without lowering the HDL (good) cholesterol .

Canola oil also contains 6% of an omega-3 fatty acid which is believed to be beneficial in preventing and treating heart disease by inhibiting blood clot formation. Whether the small amount of omega-3 in canola oil is enough to make a significant health difference is debatable, but it can't hurt.

Currently canola oil is imported from Canada and Europe and is more expensive than most other vegetable oils despite being less expensive to produce. That's because marketing geniuses know we are willing to pay more money for a product that we believe has health enhancing benefits.

Bottom line? Try it. Incorporate it into your salad dressings and other foods that require oils (minute amounts, please). Keep your total fat to 30% or less of your total diet. And keep your eyes open for new products!

ON THE ROAD AGAIN

Here in the Pacific Northwest, where I live most of the year, it is a long time between cities when one travels primarily by car, so I often find myself facing a long drive to fulfill a business commitment. Last week as I set off on a four and a half hour trip I became aware of how much my travel preparations have changed since twenty years ago when I was traveling with two young children. Back then there were no tape decks and few radio stations that satisfactorily entertained all of us. My memory and creativity were regularly challenged as I told the kids real and made-up stories and encouraged them to sing along to musical classics like "I've Been Workin' on the Railroad" and "Eensy Weensy Spider." In those days the cooler was stocked with Oreo cookies, peanut butter sandwiches, candy bars and other "treats". I am embarassed to admit I used these high in fat treats to bribe them to be more patient between the many bathroom stops and park breaks.

These days I usually travel alone. I entertain myself with a small portable library of musical and instructional tapes chosen to suit any mood that may come my way. Instead of candy bars and bologna sandwiches, now my cooler is filled with fresh fruit and bagels and non-fat yogurt. I used to think bottled water was ridiculous. Now I carry an icy jugful of it.

For those of you who travel with children, Portland newspaper columnist Kaye Van Valkenburg offers some additional suggestions. She takes "Wee Sing" and Raffi tapes for her three and six year old offspring and uses library books-on-tape for additional entertainment. She also carries air-popped popcorn and "juice in a box" and a supply of "real food" snack treats, including prunes, "to help the travelers maintain a sunny disposition."

Last but not least, I no longer drive with my destination as the sole focus of the trip. I give myself extra time to follow any side road or stop at any park my heart desires. And most of all, as I travel down the road, I try to rejoice in my successful new lifestyle—and not wish that I'd figured it out earlier.

HOW MUCH WEIGHT CAN YOU CARRY?

In chapter three of this book you learned I am an advocate of getting rid of the height/weight/body frame charts and using body fat percentages to compute a realistic weight goal. If you know your body fat percentage and subsequently your pounds of fat and pounds of non-fat (or lean) you can have some fun with a formula originated by fitness guru Covert Bailey. Bailey's formula calculates the amount of weight his workshop participants should be able to carry in their back packs. It also works for computing grocery bag weight or pounds of children or gravel or anything else you need to move from one place to another. Bailey says you should be able to carry a maximum weight that is one-half of your lean body weight.

Suppose at 120 pounds you are 25% fat. That means you have 30 pounds of fat and 90 pounds of non-fat, or lean. If you are familiar with how heavy 45 pounds is (1/2 of 90 pounds) you are probably groaning and saying forget it. But wait! You are already carrying your own weight, so to speak. There is already 30 pounds of body fat in that imaginary pack. Subtract that from the 45 pounds and your actual pack requirement is reduced to fifteen pounds. Now there is a good deal! A 120 pound, 25% fat person should be able to carry fifteen pounds of anything for a substantial period of time.

But will you do me a favor? Follow safe "lifting" guidelines by distributing it so you don't put pressure on any one muscle group. In the meantime, you have a new tool for living the Lowfat Lifestyle!

STOP!

I'll bet you thought you were only half way through the book. You may have turned the page wondering what you would read about next.

You *are* half way through the book and you *are* finished with Nutrition Nuggets and More. And, you are *not* finished. If you turn the page, you will discover the rest of the book is upside down. How could the publisher have made such a serious error?

There are no mistakes. Everything happens for a reason.

When people begin to make changes in the way they choose food or exercise things begin to happen to them. They discover more than their eating and movement habits have changed. *They* have changed and there are new beginnings in other areas of their lives. They discover their life has changed. There is a story there.

So, turn the book over and begin again. You will read about these Changes-The Rest of the Story.

CHANGES

THE REST OF THE STORY

BY RONDA GATES

TABLE OF CONTENTS

INTRODUCTION

Life is a process. We are ever changing. When life feels static we say we are in a rut. When the rut lasts a long time we talk about repeating self-defeating behaviors.

Most people who come to hear me lecture say they want to be motivated–to move out of their rut. I remind them that they are already motivated–that is why they are there. They are, in fact, looking for the practical tools to help them maintain their commitment to change.

I teach them what I know about how to choose food and exercise and we explore ways it will enhance their mental and physical well being. They make choices about which of these ideas they are comfortable using and experiment with new ways to put into practice what they have learned. At the same time, with their input, we begin to notice how and why their long standing self-defeating behaviors reoccur, establish a supportive team, and absorb and integrate new learnings. They make small changes. In time these small changes slowly turn these behaviors around and add up to a big change–a lifestyle change.

As we gather in support of one another trust and rapport becomes the framework in which these stories are shared. We discover that on one level or another these experiences are startingly similar.

The stories that follow are composites of some of those experiences. Like other readers if you recognize a part of yourself there it is probably because they are experiences that could happen or have happened to many of us. I share them because in recognizing our patterns in others I believe we come to the awareness that we are not alone. Enjoy the reading and begin your own noticing.

AFFIRMATIONS

It was the first session of a new weight management class. "I'd like each of you to introduce yourself by the name you would like to be called in class, and add a self-descriptive comment that will help us remember who you are," I said. As an example I introduced myself. "I'm Ronda and you'll probably remember my southern drawl."

A young looking woman volunteered to start. "I'm Jennifer and I have nine children ages nine to nineteen." We all admitted we were stunned and agreed it would be difficult to forget that fact. We turned to the next participant. "I'm Rebecca and my hobby is roses. I have over 100 varieties in my garden including a prize winner from last year's Rose Festival competition." Since Pat was wearing a rose dress we knew we would remember her. Would she be willing to dress in rosy hues throughout the course? We all laughed and moved on. "My name is Diana," the next participant said, with a shy smile. "I'm a klutz!" She then showed us an ugly leg bruise she got when her foot slipped through a grate. "I do this kind of stuff all the time. I'm just a walking disaster!" I smiled. I knew Diana was going to see a big change in her life in the next weeks.

The introductions continued and I gave the students an overview of the class including a list of the things I was going to ask them to do as part of changing their behavior processes. I started with affirmations. "How many of you have experience with affirmations?" I asked. As usual everyone had heard of affirmations but only three of the twelve women had used them. "Well, regardless of what you think about them", I said, "I want each of you to make one affirmation about any reasonable part of your life you would like to change for the better." The usual shuffling followed.

Begin your affirmation with the word, "I." This is a strong statement of your personal power.

I remembered my own reaction the first time I was asked to use affirmations. I found myself feeling moderately uncomfortable and heard a voice in my head saying, "Oh no, not this stuff! This is stupid." My teacher challenged me in the same way I was now challenging my class. She gave me some guidelines.

Begin your affirmation with the word, "I." This is a strong statement of your personal power.

Always affirm in the now. Instead of "I am getting better and better every day," say, "I am better."

Affirm with "I have" rather than the "I need" or "I want": "I have poise and confidence in every situation." " I have good balance."

Omit the word "should" from affirmations. It's a dangerous word anytime. Instead of "I should...," say, "I do."

The words "no," "non," "not," and "never" are negative words in affirmations. "I am not clumsy," or "I no longer fall down," or "I never fall" are all reminders of a powerful part of you that you want to change–but they are negative, defeating reminders. A more useful choice is "I am poised and confident and have steady feet." "I have excellent balance."

The words "hope," wish," and "try" are illusory. Have you ever "tried" to pick up a set of car keys? You reach out and you pick them up! It is much easier, it takes less energy to do things than to "try to" or "want to" or "need to" do them. Instead of trying to get over my fear of heights or hoping it would go away I climbed stairs on the outside of a local seven story warehouse and said, "I am comfortable climbing higher with each step." My heart was pounding but after many repetitions of this exercise my fear diminished.

Anytime you slip into old self-abusive speaking patterns add the words, "up until now." For example, if Diana noticed herself saying, "I'm a klutz," the added phrase would take the power from the negative affirmation.

After you have created your affirmation repeat it to yourself several times. If it feels comfortable to you, you have chosen well. Most people adjust the wording of their affirmation several times before it feels "right".

Remember the old saying, "Be careful of what you wish for. You may get it?" When you make an affirmation, you get it. It is a message that reaches your semi-conscious or subconscious mind; many studies have shown that a message that reaches that part of your mind rings true despite what the conscious mind knows.

As instructed, Diana wrote and then read her affirmation at least once every morning and every evening. It read, "I move gracefully and confidently through my day." She recorded it several times on a cassette tape as an "I" statement and asked her husband to do the same as a "you" statement to her. She played the tape daily. Soon she found herself automatically thinking the affirmation in her head. And, later, her experience duplicated mine. She noticed a subtle change. She was walking with pride and confidence. "I don't know and I don't care why or how it works," Diana reported seven weeks later. "I'm a convert! Watch out world! Here I come!"

A VICTIM
OF ANGER

Linda wanted to meet me at noon. Her schedule was so tight; "only the lunch hour" would work for her. I agreed to hold our individual consultation at the club that hosts my weight management class. Linda was not a member of the club, but was prepared to pay the surcharge that would be necessary to attend the class there. I had been consulting with her on an individual basis for a couple of weeks before the group experience got started, focusing on her history and the problems she felt were specific to herself. She had made some small changes and for the first time was maintaining her weight without feeling like she was dieting.

When I arrived at the club I was given a message that Linda would be about fifteen minutes late. I geared myself up for the part that would be difficult for me-closing the appointment at the appropriate time despite the fact she had not received her full hour. I filled a cup with ice water, read a newspaper and waited for her.

At 12:20 I was paged. to the front desk. Linda was there and she was angry. When she had asked for me the woman at the desk had told her, "There is no one here by that name." I acknowledged her feelings and asked Linda if she would like to go on the patio-the day was one of Portland's best and the seating was appropriate for a private conversation. "No," she replied, "I want to get something to eat. If I don't eat now I may not get to eat for the rest of the day. I have a real full schedule that goes through the evening."

As we headed for the dining room I told Linda that the club had a policy of exchanging no cash. Since she had not yet paid her surcharge she was not entitled to club privileges of ordering and charging a meal. There was, however, a possibility that with the exact change she could bargain with the kitchen crew for something to eat. I sat back to watch what would happen.

Linda marched to the counter. She was greeted by a cheery waitress who asked what Linda would like. A lengthy conversation followed with Linda looking more and more bristly and the waitress holding her tongue in the best tradition of making the customer right.

Ten minutes later Linda returned with a salad. She was really angry! She could not believe it was that much trouble to get something to eat. She seemed near tears as she expressed her frustration at how she had to jump through hoops to be able to eat what she wanted when she wanted.

An opportunity had presented itself. After some supportive acknowledgement of her difficulty I asked her what some of these other experiences were. "My husband doesn't help at all," she said. "He does all the grocery shopping and when I ask him to bring me something special he always comes home with the wrong thing. Last week I asked him to buy that breast of chicken that's only 30 calories a slice. He came home with a whole chicken breast. I'd wanted the sliced chicken breast. I had no idea it came in whole pieces. You wouldthink he'd have known what I wanted."

I asked Linda why she didn't shop for her own food. "My husband's checkbook is the one that is used for food. If I buy food with my checkbook it will screw everything up." She said she did not go with him because she didn't have time.

Weight management is always tied up with things other than eating.

Linda is a victim of her own creation. She has expectations of other people and places that she does not express, then becomes angry when she doesn't get what she wants. Projecting her own way of doing things onto someone else, she assumes everything will work out all right for her. When it doesn't she becomes a "victim," is no longer responsible for her perceived powerlessness and can become "justifiably" angry.

I began some active problem solving with Linda on this very issue. I pointed out that although it seemed sensible to assume she would be able to get a meal at the health club restaurant, that did not happen. I shared one of my own experiences learning about assumption. After a particularly frustrating experience a friend pointed out to me that the word "assume" breaks down to ass-u-me! Assuming makes an ass out of you and me. I encouraged Linda to note how often she makes assumptions.

From a practical point of view we looked at alternative ways she could eat lunch on a regular basis, since I knew her schedule was not going to change. Linda was not ready to look at the role her overbooked day played in helping her avoid some painful issues. Since her consulting work takes her to the same businesses on a weekly basis I asked her to track her travels. She was to become aware of restaurants she believed would serve the foods that were in keeping with the lifestyle changes she was trying to make. She would have to take the time to visit a few of them, ask to see a menu and find out if she could place telephone orders to go.

We also explored ways she could carry foods with her that were fulfilling and satisfying alternatives if she did not find time to go to a restaurant. She agreed one of the new thermos bags or a cooler would be handy in her car. It could be filled with bagels, non fat yogurt, cut fresh fruit, low fat cheese and a variety of refreshing drinks.

I also suggested that, if her husband was going to continue to take full responsibility for their food shopping, Linda might have to make the time to go with him at least once to show him which foods she wanted. I encouraged her to save the labels off these foods, put them in plastic, and if necessary, to give him the labels as a reminder. We also decided to make a personal, very specific shopping list that she could photocopy. She could circle the items she wanted and be sure he understood what they were before he went to the market.

Mutually, Linda and I had found some alternatives to situations that were frustrating her. Her face and body relaxed slightly. When she returned two weeks later she reported that she had done her homework, had some successes and was feeling hopeful she could continue to problem solve.

Weight management is always tied up with things other than eating. For Linda, it had to do with expectations and victimization and anger. Her therapist will be challenged to help her deal with those issues. In the meantime, we will continue the process of bandaiding the day to day stuff until all the pieces fall into place.

And me? At five minutes after one I told Linda it was time to bring the appointment to a close. She tried to hang on and I struggled to take care of myself. When we parted, I sighed. This time I had gotten off only ten minutes late. The previous time it had been fifteen. I was getting better too.

IT'S THE BEEF?

Thirty of us were sitting on mats in the mountain lodge where I was attending a lengthy conference. After a "free day" we felt a sense of expectancy as we each reported on what the previous day had brought our way.

When Anita "checked in" she said she had decided to stay around the lodge, walk and read, and just take it easy. Later that night when she had difficulty sleeping, she reviewed her day. Anita, who has been eating a more vegetarian diet told us how much better she had been feeling. Recently she had decided her body couldn't handle meat any more. She believed her discomfort was because she had deviated from her new eating style the day before when she had succumbed to the lunch hour craving for a hamburger (which she enjoyed). The hamburger was supplemented later that evening with a piece of pepperoni pizza her roommate brought back from her own outing. "I think it was the meat that set me off," Anita stated assertively. I struggled with the impulse to give a quick response and I succumbed. "Not the meat, it was the fat in the meat," I quipped. Everyone looked at me.

They did not understand what I was talking about. Most people do not understand this effect of dietary fat. They are not equipped with some basic knowledge about food and, having only limited information, like Anita, they often come to conclusions that may be erroneous.

The scoundrel in red meat is the fat, not the meat itself.

People often come up to me at lectures with faces glowing as they tell me about the changes they have made as they eat a more wholesome diet. "I don't eat red meat anymore," they tell me, as their halo vibrates. "Oh? What kind of meat do you eat?" I ask, "green meat or blue meat or yellow meat?" I get the same taken aback look I saw on everyone's faces when I responded to Anita.

Whether you choose to include or exclude meat in your diet is your own business. What you need to know is that the scoundrel in red meat is the fat, not the meat itself. Meat is an excellent source of top-quality protein, vitamins and minerals, especially the B vitamins and iron. When the cut of meat you choose is not lean, the price you pay for all those nutrients can be high, especially if you eat a lot of meat.

I tell my friends to brag about a diet that is free of greasy meats. I no longer eat greasy meats myself. Instead of the prime rib and sirloin steak I used to favor, I choose lean cuts of chicken, pork and beef. I also learned a long time ago to focus on vegetables and grains as the main part of my meal. Now the meat in my diet is there as a condiment.

When I am in restaurants I sometimes see people blotting their food before they eat it. I smile, knowing their health consciousness has been raised. The public is catching on to the real dangers of greasy food.

BULIMICS
WHO CRY

I jumped when my office phone rang at 8:30 one night. It was Jenni, a 26-year-old student in my twelve week weight management class. Jenni was a recovering bulimic and she was often frantic about her weight.

Bulimia is a life-threatening disease that is manifested by alternating bouts of eating and purging. The most common purge is vomiting but the use of laxative, diuretics and exercise are other ways people who struggle with eating disorders get rid of calories they believe will turn to body fat.

Jeni was not overweight. Most bulimics are not–they just see themselves that way. Jeni was no exception. So, although she has been purge free for six months each time she looked in the mirror she still struggled with her distorted image.

Jeni was able to sustain her effort to continue the personal introspection necessary to live more healthy because she had the professional support of a competent therapist and the personal support of a group of friends eager to see her suceed. She had "come clean" with her family when she told them that she spent most of her day sneaking food, then vomiting.

I met Jenni when she decided she needed more information on how to balance her new lifestyle. Now she exercised regularly and was learning how to make better food choices in the framework of foods she enjoyed. She waffled on her new eating plan periodically, but said even when she ate too much she didn't vomit. She took advantage of the permission granted by her therapist, her sponsor in Overeater's Anonymous and me to call any time she felt threatened by her old habits. That got her through difficult moments until she had time, in therapy, to work on her issues more deeply.

Jenni was glad to hear my voice. She wanted to come over to my office. I often stop by my office after an evening class to wind down my day. I agreed it was okay for her to drop in. She arrived looking sheepish. "I feel so bad calling you at this late hour," she told me. "No problem," I responded. Our agreement was that she could call anytime, and if I was free we would get together. Tonight I was, quite honestly, delighted to see her. She was a walking success story!

Comforting our loved ones
has its place, but not when it
prevents experiencing the grief
that accompanies all endings and is
required to move on with our life.

As Jenni sat down she said, "I feel out of control. I don't want to eat or vomit or do anything crazy, but I seem to cry at the least little thing." Tears welled up in her eyes as she told me, "I feel so sensitive. Everything triggers tears." I hummed inside. Jenni had a lot to cry about. She had been a smoker since the age of thirteen. When she whipped that habit at 21 she began drinking too much. When she realized she was drinking more than she wanted, she quit cold but found herself gaining weight as she turned to food for solace. Since she worked and went to school it was hard for her to find time to exercise so she started vomiting to get rid of the calories that she could not "work" off.

Jenni is experiencing recovery from what is described as cross addictions. When she stopped using cigarettes, then alcohol, then food every time she felt uncomfortable and needed a "fix", she found herself face to face with a full range of emotions that were scary.

I have learned that there are always good reasons for tears. Most of us have not been able to grieve the losses in our life. When we feel sad other people feel uncomfortable, and they find all kinds of ways to console us. Comforting our loved ones has its place, but not when it prevents experiencing the grief that accompanies all endings and is required to move on with our life.

Jenni's tears turned to sobs and she soon found herself in touch with that part of her missing her lost opportunities of the past fifteen years. I was proud of her. I rarely meet someone as young as Jenni who is willing to come to grips with their disease–and bulimia is certainly a disease. I also empathized with her pain and knew that when this crying spell was over she would have pieced together yet another part of her story and could move on with her life.

After a short twenty minute cry Jenni was feeling better. In fact, it was not long before we were drinking tea and laughing over a funny experience she had at work. "I can't believe how much better I feel," Jenni said. We talked a little longer about the joy of life on the mend and Jenni agreed she would hold on to this post-sorrow moment as a light at the end of the next painful phase of healing growth that would surely come her way.

14 Changes

It has been two years since Jenni joined my class. She is still a success story. She is graduating from nursing school next month. Lots of my stories have happy endings!

FURY FITS

Jo Ann was feeling confident! The weight management class she was attending was in its fifth week and when we met for a counselling appointment she seemed on track and comfortable with her goals.

Jo Ann is a graphic artist who left a high powered job with a major firm to work out of her home. That gave her the time she needed to focus on her recovery from compulsive eating and still generate enough income to support her. Jo Ann's therapist had given her my name as a resource for some perspective on how to choose foods more wisely. The work Jo Ann and I had done together had helped considerably, but her craving for sweets often overcame her. Periodically she had succumbed to a sweet tooth which often resulted in her eating more fat than we had allotted for her diet. At our previous appointment she re-committed to noticing what was going on when that happened.

"You seem happy," I told Jo Ann as we sat down.

"I can't believe it," she replied exuberantly, "I haven't been craving sweets for six days and I've been able to stick to my diet without any difficulty. In fact, it no longer seems like a diet at all. I just eat when I'm hungry and follow the guidelines we set up a couple of weeks ago. I'm eating foods I enjoy and don't have any cravings I can't deal with on a moment to moment basis."

I had to know more. "Anything you can key into?" I inquired. "Yes," Jo Ann said. "On hindsight it seems simpler than I thought. You know I've been working with my therapist on the relationship between food and my moods, and I came to the awareness a couple of months ago that I crave food when I don't want to deal with my feelings. I've had that awareness for a couple months, but until last week I hadn't fully been able to act on it."

"Last week I had a breakthrough. I was feeling really stressed and wanted to eat all the time. When I looked at what was going on, I realized I was on overload. I couldn't see any way out of the responsibilities I'd chosen to undertake and my assistant seemed to be getting in my way more than helping me. As the week went on my jaw got tighter and tighter and I realized that I had been 'locking' my jaw instead of saying the things I needed to say."

"Since I'm still not skilled in the way I confront people, I was afraid to try, so I stayed with that feeling a while and I realized there was some underlying anger that had nothing to do with my secretary. My therapist has encouraged me to allow myself the time to let it evolve, and soon I was in a full blown rage attack."

"I have a bunch of cardboard tubes I've been using to hit the couch when I get angry and they were ripped to shreds in five minutes. Suddenly I was wishing I had the bataka that's in my therapist's office. I felt almost crazy, and the tears and noise and anger all combined into a crescendo of my fury. I kept hearing my gremlin voice saying 'Stop the noise!' and

'Don't be so loud!' and all the other messages that come into my head anytime I get into this feelings stuff."

"But, I told those old voice messages to go to hell, and pretty soon I was exhausted and felt the process had passed. I slept like a log that night. When my secretary arrived the next day I admitted to her I had some difficulty with the work she was doing for me and we worked out a plan that served us both."

"I haven't been eating compulsively since. In fact, I went away for the weekend with a group of friends and had very little difficulty staying on my eating program. It was easy to avoid overeating the few sweets that someone brought along. I allowed myself to revel in those successes and here I am today, feeling I have it licked."

> My personal experience
> and those of my clients
> have shown me that turning to food
> instead of dealing with our feelings
> is so ingrained in us
> it is hard to catch it every time.

Jo Ann does not have it licked. She does have a great success under her belt, some new behaviors that worked well for her. Happily for her, she gave herself a lot of credit for her "work", and if she is lucky she will be able to hold onto that experience for a while and tap into it the next time she is headed towards an eating binge. My personal experience and those of my clients have shown me that turning to food instead of dealing with our feelings is so ingrained in us it is hard to catch it every time.

I'm several years into my own recovery from compulsive eating and still have stressful periods when I realize I have been eating mindlessly. But, it is getting better. Each day I count the successes–including expressing a full range of feelings I used to avoid. I like the self esteem that comes from knowing who I am, what I want and need, and my increasing ability to stay with myself on a day to day basis.

Jo Ann and I discussed the need to plan for future episodes. If she stays in touch with the relationship between her desire to eat and her feelings during her latest experience she will lick it again, and then again. And in time she will accumulate, as I have, increasingly more successes than relapses.

I pointed out to Jo Ann that every client I have ever worked with has her own particular pace for putting a new lifestyle in place. Some clients seem to get on track quickly and others have been working on it for a couple of years. Even slow starters' are a lot better than they were when we began working together and we make a point of reminding ourselves of that regularly.

Sometimes I am asked if there is a class for "retards", and I offer reassurance that no one is a retard once you have made a commitment to a new lifestyle. Many of those folk who have been doing their lifestyle work for a couple of years check in with me on a periodic basis to readjust goals and to update me on their progress. These are wonderful visits for me and I am looking forward to more of them with Jo Ann.

MARIE
CHANGES JOBS

I expected my friend Marie to be floating on the ceiling. She had just been accorded one of the highest honors in her profession, election to the presidency of her professional organization. However, when we met to work on a project, she seemed nervous. Prior to leaving her office for our meeting her boss told her she was one of three candidates eligible for promotion to the vice presidency of the company where she had been working the last six years. Attaining the new position would be fulfillment of many of her personal and professional goals, including being the first woman to rise to such a high level in a profession that had, heretofore, been dominated by men.

"Ronda, I've been under so much pressure the past few months with the projects I'm working on, I haven't had the time I need to exercise regularly and I've put on about fifteen pounds," Marie said. "I'm afraid I won't get this new position because it has a high public profile, and I'm not attractive enough. How can I get this weight off fast?"

Marie is almost six feet tall. She is a striking brunette who carries her weight well and I did not note much of a difference from the last time I saw her. But I was not going to discount her feelings. She also confided that her "love life" was next to nothing. "But I guess that's okay," she said. "At this weight I don't want anyone to see or touch my body anyway."

Whether we gained weight slowly or quickly we used food as a substance to nurture ourselves.

Marie's predicament was not news to me. As a lifestyle teacher and counsellor I meet many women who believe their weight is a primary obstacle in their personal development path so they are constantly on a diet. I told Marie of my theory that those of us who practice yo-yo dieting for so many years are, in effect, practicing a less extreme form of the binge-purge cycle.

Whether we gain weight slowly or quickly we use food as a substance to nurture ourselves. The inevitable increase in weight fulfills the binge part of the cycle. When we ultimately become disgusted with ourselves, we turn to the latest crash diet, including sometimes near-starvation levels of eating (or not eating) that fulfill the purge component of the process. As I have spent more time with clients we have discovered a number of underlying issues that precipitate this form of "nourishment" and subsequent punishment. I am particularly surprised when I hear, from one client after another, how each has suffered some form of physical, emotional or sexual abuse in their younger years.

Marie seemed thoughtful then she said, "I don't remember any form of abuse when I was growing up. I was the only girl of four children and clearly my father's favorite. Dad was proud of me, especially the way I looked. In fact, one of the reasons I've always taken pride in caring for myself is because it always pleased him so much when I looked pretty. I remember when I was growing up, how he would tell me that if I stayed beautiful and thin and well dressed I would always have lots of men around me and would never have to worry about being lonely. He said that if I got fat and ugly no one would want me. He even used to weigh me every Friday so we could be sure that...."

Marie's words trailed off into silence. I did not have to tell her what was going through my mind. Weighed every Friday! And, perhaps praised if the numbers on the scale were lower and berated if they were higher than Marie's–and her father's goal.

Marie's eyes filled with tears as she realized that it had been emotionally and, yes, sexually abusive for her father to weigh her every week–and to associate her physical weight with her desirability, not only to her father but to the men in her future. By realizing and acknowledging this Marie had taken the first scary step of a journey that would open some doors that explain her preoccupation with her image.

Marie told me of a period in her life when she had been a borderline anorexic, followed by years of binging and purging that ended when her workaholic career became the addictive process that took her focus away from the addictive substance, food. Now, under the stress and pressure of her job she had returned to food to avoid dealing with the discomfort her new lifestyle had created in her life. She was afraid she would also return to the unhealthy binging that had once been part of her life; she wanted to get rid of the excess weight-fast.

Marie knew she could crash diet her way to a thinner appearance but it would not be the way to a leaner body. There is no fast way to lose fat weight. No matter how fast it comes on, fat cannot disappear at a rate of more than about two pounds a week.

I asked Marie if she wanted to continue to go through the yo-yo pattern that had been her history or was she willing to recommit to regular exercise and learn how to eat more healthily–for the rest of her life. I reminded her that in her career she had been willing to make time for extra-curricular courses that had improved her work options. Now she could focus that same energy toward extra-curricular course work that would improve her lifestyle options.

Marie agreed. She gave herself permission to set aside time to learn how to choose foods with more savvy and to return to the active lifestyle she loved. With the help of a compassionate support group she explored the issues that precipitated her addictive lifestyle. Slowly and steadily, she shed the extra pounds. She did not get the job she wanted. Instead, she found a new position in an organization where she was able to pace herself in a way that enabled her to live more in touch with her day-to-day process. And, no longer controlled by external referenting to others, she came to love herself well enough to glow from within.

Last week Marie called to ask me if I was going to be busy March 10, the day she is getting married to a man who shares her desire to live a day to day lifestyle.

PANIC ATTACKS

This appointment with Peggy was not going to be easy. I had known Peggy a long time. She was one of the first women I met when I moved to Minnesota and joined a neighborhood tennis league. We became casual friends who shared child-rearing, gardening and redecorating experiences. She was a devoted mother, an active volunteer and an avid gardener and bird watcher. Peggy literally glowed when she talked about her birds and often spent joyful hours in various sanctuaries tracking migratory habits and investigating nests. We had lost touch over the years, but our paths crossed at a concert one night when I was working in Minneapolis and she was delighted to hear my work had evolved into weight management.

Peggy was desperate to lose weight. That was not a surprise. Peggy had always struggled with her weight. Her longest period of success was when she worked with a dietitian, but in time she had gained it all back. The intervening years had not been kind and I saw in her eyes the hope that maybe this time she had discovered true help. She found the behavior element of the course work appealing. Like most of my clients who have played the yo-yo diet game for years, Peggy "knew a lot about food," and "what she had to do," but she did not know why she kept compromising her success.

I felt apprehensive. Peggy and I had exchanged at least a half-dozen phone calls before the first class, and she told me about a series of major illnesses and accompanying life changes since I had last seen her. She was now suffering from depression, panic attacks, compulsive eating and crying spells. She had been to many physicians in an effort to "get better," and had "tried everything" including a trip to the Mayo Clinic. Peggy was unable to tolerate anti-depressants. In fact, she said she experienced little or no relief from any of the mental or physical health professionals she had seen. Estrogen made her feel better but contributed to the extra pounds that made her worst fears of the past ten years come true. She was visibly over fat. Her lengthy yo-yo diet history indicated that metabolically she would be a challenging client.

Peggy is an adult child of an alcoholic mother and an emotionally abusive father. She also told me she had been sexually abused by an uncle. As we talked she poured out stories that would horrify the friends she so desperately tried to keep a happy face for all her life. I knew I could not help Peggy resolve her psychological and emotional issues. I also believed the class material could make her a more savvy consumer and allow her to make wiser choices when she did overeat. I accepted her into the program. During the first class she admitted she was amazed at my focus on fat instead of calories and delighted that I had no list of "good" or "bad" foods. I served frozen yogurt as a snack. It was the first time Peggy had eaten it because "it has so much sugar!" She listened to my introduction about the behavior part of the class, but her face indicated she was looking for easier answers than I would offer.

When Peggy arrived for the individual conference we greeted one another with a hug. I could feel the fear in her body and see the sadness on her face. She was depressed. She told me,

"I just *have* to lose weight. I hate myself. If I were just thin...."
She started to cry. Through her tears she once again shared
her fears about the ongoing crying spells and panic attacks.

She told me she had been in a grocery store to purchase some
baked chicken at a deli. When she returned to her car a panic
attack began. She ripped open the chicken, ate it all and
immediately felt better. "Isn't that crazy?" she asked, as tears
welled again in her eyes. I longed to comfort her, but sat still,
knowing she needed to let out feelings that had been stuffed
inside her for years. Peggy had a lot to cry about and until she
did it I was certain her underlying emotions would return
again and again. But Peggy couldn't "let go." She pulled
herself together saying, "I'm so embarrassed. I'm sick of this
crying. How long is this craziness going to go on? Isn't three
years enough!?"

Is Peggy crazy? I'm not a therapist, but my long experience
managing my own recovery as an adult child of a dysfunctional family, and as a recovering overeater, as well as experiences with my clients, has given me lots of insight into the
origins of our self-defeating behaviors, including how we
view ourselves when we are engaged in them. There are so
many facets to Peggy's "disease" that I can't begin to address
them all here. But in that one outburst she summed it up.
When Peggy is fearful she eats to fill that empty hole inside
that can be experienced as any or all of a full range of
emotions, from sadness to full blown panic. She expressed
what she hoped was the easy answer–that if she became thin
everything would be alright. Like many of my clients, Peggy
hasn't realized that changing the wrapping does not change
what's inside.

Peggy also expressed another crucial piece of her puzzle; her
compulsive eating had been translated into a self-hating
comment, reinforcing the self image that she could not help
but acquire in her alcoholic and abusive family of origin–that
she is no good. Peggy also showed how skilled she has
become in turning off her feelings. She has "cried long

enough" and doesn't want to "feel that way anymore". But, until she chooses to work her way through the anger and grieve her losses they will return again. Until she has *really* had enough she will probably continue to look for bandaids to put on her symptoms.

Children from alcoholic or any dysfunctional environments share most of the characteristics Peggy exemplifies, to a greater or lesser degree. I have not met one person who struggles with weight who doesn't ultimately discover there was dysfunction in his or her family of origin.

Sadly, Peggy's time is running out. Although she told me she is willing to try anything, and despite her family history of dysfunction and her own compulsive overeating, she turned down an invitation to go to an Overeater's Anonymous or Adult Children of Alcoholics meeting with me. "I know my mother is an alcoholic, but I've put all that behind me now," she said. "I don't want to talk about it and I don't want to sit around and listen to other people talk about it," she insisted.

I don't know if ACA or OA can help Peggy. That's where I found the support to admit I was powerless over my addictive patterns (including eating), and where I began a journey that has helped me live more functionally. As it was, Peggy's last meeting resulted in another impasse for her. My class was being held in a health club. Non-members were welcome to attend but had to pay a 50% discounted surcharge for full use of the club facilities during the ten week course. Peggy decided she couldn't afford it. I knew better. I was going to ask for more than she was ready to give and she intuitively sensed it. Once again she could be a victim of circumstances beyond her control, and the club could be the bad guy.

I called Peggy every week until I left Minnesota. She's still struggling with compulsive eating, depression and panic attacks. She is also still defending herself and her decision to leave the class, wishing "it" would go away. It won't.

SHIFTS

I liked my appointments with Sharon. She sparkles. Sharon is a successfully recovering bulimic. She had been purge-free more eight months, managing her diet and exercise in a wholesome way, and her skin, hair, face and body had resumed a more healthful appearance. We were getting together to run her current food choices through my computer and see if she needed to make any additional changes.

As Sharon settled into the chair next to me her eyes welled with tears. She twisted her mouth, seemed embarrassed and said, "I'm so sensitive these days. It seems like everything makes me want to cry." I asked if something specific was bothering her today and she said she had been thinking about a long term friendship that was fading from her life.

Sharon and Mary had played golf, gone to parties, shopped and talked kids together for many years. Mary was involved in lots of activities and led a very full life. Sharon described her as a "people pleaser". In the process of her own "recovery" Sharon realized that their friendship was lopsided. Sharon was the one who called Mary every day and Sharon was the one who made all the plans for the events they went to together. Because "Mary was so busy", Mary never called Sharon or invited her to parties or arranged the family outings they shared.

When Sharon thought about it, she realized she had lots of busy and needy friends. She also became aware of her role in taking care of some of the—especially Mary. Sharon had compromised her own self-care by allowing herself to keep busy and focus outside herself–avoiding the time necessary to deal with her own issues.

With encouragement from her therapist Sharon began to make changes. Next time she was with Mary Sharon explained that in the past, because she knew Mary had so much to do she had always made the arrangements for them to get together. Now Sharon wanted Mary to share some responsibility for the friendship by occasionally initiating some activities and phone calls. "Sure," Mary agreed. "No problem."

Happily, Sharon sat back and waited. A couple of days went by and she did not hear from Mary. The days stretched to a week, then two weeks. Sharon longed to pick up the phone, but did not. Their paths crossed at parties where her friend was always quite cheery, but the time they spent together dwindled to nothing. Mary always shared lots of stories about how her summer was going and the many activities in her life, activities she had formerly done with Sharon and was now doing with other women. Sharon missed her friend. She finally confessed to Mary that she was sad that they no longer spent so much time together, that Mary had never called her and that it felt like Mary no longer cared enough about the friendship to provide her share.

Mary reacted as Sharon expected. She told Sharon that nothing was wrong, she felt fine about the relationship and had just been "too busy." She said Sharon was "just imagining things." Sharon's inside voice told her this wasn't true. She did not know who to believe; maybe she was crazy.

I had been the caretaker in most of my relationships

It was easy for me to be empathetic with Sharon. When I made a decision to change the way I lived my life I had a similar experience. Like Sharon I realized that I had been the caretaker in most of my relationships-a responsibility I had gladly assumed and one that kept me busy and filled my life with many friends. When I asked my family and friends to share the responsibility for the time we spent together, some of them did. Sadly, many of them did not. Like Sharon, I called some of them and, like Sharon, they told me I was crazy, everything was "fine." But they still did not call. When we crossed paths they acted as if nothing was wrong and for awhile I doubted myself. It was good to feel the old closeness until I realized "the old closeness" was "feeling scared." I had felt scared with many of my friends. I began to wonder if I had inherently known back then that I would lose their friendship if I did not do 99% of the work. That was why I felt scared; I was desperate to hold on to those friendships. I have no doubt those people cared about me. But they liked the caretaking Ronda. And the sad fact is our friendship was not valuable enough for them to make the 50% effort necessary to sustain it.

I shared my experiences with Sharon and told her that, for me, changing and growing meant suffering some loss. Most people want their world to remain static. Even the people who loved me and were happy to see me move out of a dysfunctional environment were not comfortable with the new me. I was different, and they felt it as a challenge. I was not imposing on them, but they felt threatened. After all, when friends saw me experiencing some of the pain of growth, many of them encouraged me (and Sharon) to "forget all this stuff if it makes you unhappy."

Whenever I start a new weight management class I spend a lot of time reminding everyone that their most supportive loved ones may not, ultimately, like the changes they will want to make. I see life as a mobile. I am just one part of it. When I change my place in the mobile, throwing it off balance, others must accept my new position or make their own adjustments to be comfortable in the new shape the mobile assumes. It is not easy.

I encouraged Sharon to work through her grief. I was willing to be there if she needed a shoulder to cry on, and told her so. As it happened our meeting was a gift. Sharon lived less than a mile from me and we had both been hoping new friends would come into our lives to replace the ones we had moved beyond. Sharon and I became friends.

THERESA'S
COOKIE MONSTER

Theresa was having a devil of a time sticking to her weight management program. She was maintaining her daily exercise by alternating long evening walks with early morning aerobic exercise. It was her eating program that was testing her determination to change her lifestyle.

Theresa jokingly describes herself as a cookie monster. As we discussed her food options early in the weight management course, she decided she could easily handle a 20% fat diet with a daily allotment of 30 grams of fat. Since she liked fresh fruits, vegetables and high-fiber low-grain breads she was satisfied using fat-free yogurt as a base for her salad dressings, and vegetable sauces. She chose to eat low fat fish and chicken for her meat choices, low fat cheese for sandwiches and snacks. She was not willing to give up bakery cookies which to her surprise, contained 5 grams of fat apiece.

Everything had been ticking along just fine and Theresa had been losing about two pounds of fat per week for the last month. With another 11 pounds to go until she reached a realistic weight goal her emotional problems had reared their ugly head and were getting in the way of her commitment to keep the fat out of her diet.

The cookies were the problem, she explained.

At first Theresa "did" the cookies by stopping at the bakery after work, the time when she craved cookies most. She purchased three, ate one immediately and saved the remaining two for a dessert and snack later in the evening.

Then, one morning, she craved the cookies and stopped to purchase and eat them on the way to work. By evening, Theresa was in the grip of her usual habit and bought cookies again. When she talked to me she admitted she was eating cookies morning and evening and snacking on some candy in between. That, combined with two weeks when she had slept late instead of attending a 6:30 a.m. exercise class, had resulted in a two week period that left her with a clear awareness that she was slipping.

I asked her if anything unusual was going on in her life. She could not identify anything in particular until I inquired about her children. Both were college age and had returned to their out-of-state schools. Theresa also realized this month would have been the 25th anniversary of a marriage that had ended one year ago. She said the date had passed without her remembering it, and she was, quite honestly, surprised.

I knew that Theresa's sister, whom she had not seen in six years, was planning to visit and wondered if that had brought up any issues. "Oh, something came up for her and she was unable to make the trip", Theresa told me. "That must have been disappointing," I replied. "Yes, but she couldn't help it," Theresa said.

I asked Theresa to think about the times she went to purchase the cookies. What could have satisfied her as much as the cookies? She answered surprisingly quickly, Company."

Lights went on and puzzle pieces fell into place. "Do you mean that with company youd could have avoided the cookies?" "Absolutely", she replied.

Loneliness and loss are underlying issues in many self defeating behaviors around food.

We had a window through which to explore Theresa's issues.

Loneliness and loss are underlying issues in many self-defeating behaviors around food. As children, when lonely, we often received food to make us feel better. When we suffered sadness and disappointment over usual and un-usual losses, food was often offered to us to help take away the pain. How could our later relationship with food be any different? Our society equates food with love.

My early memory of the death of a close relative is of how stunned I was by the amount of food that came into the house. I figured out that bringing mountains of food was peoples' way to show others they cared. Even the forced gaiety of the mourning period, (the Irish call it a wake) revolved around good food and insisting that everyone eat.

It has become "normal" to turn to food, especially foods we like and that nurture us, when we get lonely as adults. That was what was happening to Theresa.

But what to do? I told her that for the next few days the support elements of her program were going to be impor-tant. First she needed to deal with her sadness and loneliness, to feel it and process it. Her therapist could help her there; I insisted that Theresa bring her into the picture on this issue.

And even if Theresa did not have the energy it was time to map out a plan to surround herself, even if only by phone, with a support team. "I don't want to bother them," she whined, ever so slightly. I took on my maternal tone. "You have my permission and their permission to call them," I told Theresa. "Do it."

The next week Theresa returned with a smile on her face. She was back on track and feeling pretty good about resolving her loneliness–this time. She said she had let herself succumb to a good cry once that week when she felt particularly lonely, and some little cries had come up at other times. She had called her program sponsor daily and they had gone to a movie together. That simple connection had been enough to get Theresa over this hump. She had also decided, on her own, to abstain from the cookies for three days–a technique that had staved off compulsive food urges in the past. During that time she used other foods for desserts and snacks, and she shared some of her ideas with us.

Now Theresa felt she, once again, had given herself some relief from her compulsive cookie-eating, and although she decided, for now, not to go back to the cookie routine, she felt it was still a choice in the future.

Old memory tapes are embedded in our brains. They urge us to return to long time habits, to sustain returning issues of loneliness and loss. Like Theresa, we have to be aware of these old tapes and *remain* aware of them, any time we make a lifestyle change.

MEETING MICHAEL AGAIN

Pat seemed nervous, but excited, when we met for a Portland waterfront lunch. I met Pat when she had joined my aerobic class. After seven years of regular exercise, confrontation of some dysfunctional eating patterns and use of the practical nutrition education tools we shared in class, she looked considerably younger than her 50 years. Our friendship had deepened when she recruited me as a volunteer for the Special Olympics. Pat's sister is mentally retarded and Pat is deeply committed to trying to improve the quality of life for these special people. Our lives also parallel one another's closely. We are both educators who turned from homemaker to career maker after our marriages ended. Even though we sometimes did not see one another for a couple months at a time, our friendship continued to evolve. We were at a point where we could "tell it like it is," and I sensed it would last a long time.

"What's up?" I asked. "Remember my friend, Michael," she began, "the fellow from Connecticut I used to see once in a while?" I nodded. "Well, I talked to him yesterday and we're going to see one another next week when I go to Washington." She smiled a little guiltily.

Michael is a vice president of one of the Fortune 500 companies. Pat and I had talked liked school girls about their relationship the past few years. Michael and Pat met when they served on the national board of a mental retardation agency, and they had worked together on many committees and national fund raisers over the years. The comradery that develops as people share work on a project provided an environment for establishing their own close friendship, and when their intense committee work ended they usually caught up on one another's lives over drinks and dinner in a fashionable restaurant.

At one of these meetings they discovered they were both separated from their spouses and had a lot more in common than their interest in mental retardation. Their evening of drinks turned into dinner, then dancing, and they ended up spending the night together. They returned to their respective communities but kept in touch, and the next few times their committee or conference work brought them together for a one or two day meeting they extended the trip and spent time hiking or biking or enjoying other active sports Michael was interested in.

A year later Pat and her husband decided they needed more than the emotionally void marriage they had shared for so long and it ended amicably. Michael, however, returned to his marriage. When he and Pat talked he told her he knew it wasn't all he deserved or wanted in a marriage, but like Pat's, it had lasted more than 25 years and the financial and emotional price he would have to pay if it ended "wasn't worth the hassle."

Pat justified her ongoing affair with a married man as part of her experimentation with life as a single woman. She found herself attracted to strong, charming, bright men. Although she maintained her intermittent relationship with Michael, she had a couple of affairs with other charismatic men who "weren't interested in settling down." In time she found herself committed to "a terrific guy" who "validated" her growing professional life. She had met him when she worked as a consultant with his company. She knew she was "good for him" too. He had been divorced for seven years but had never settled into another committed relationship. She knew that if given the chance she could make it work for them. Although they did not live together they spent a lot of time working and traveling together.

She had a reputation for being especially helpful to powerful women who seemed to have it all together, but did not.

But after a year Pat had to admit she could not make it work. She found herself choosing to move out of still another relationship which had been emotionally empty for her. When she had expressed her needs, although not very assertively, she found the commitment was one-sided. She was unable to meet what she was forced to acknowledge was a powerfully strong need to "belong to someone."

Pat found a dynamic therapist. She had a reputation for being especially helpful to powerful women who seem to have it all together, but do not. With her therapist's help Pat came to the awareness that it was a self esteem issue. She had been looking outside of herself for validation of her work and her relationships. She realized she had been willing to compromise her own wants and needs and negotiate for less than what she wanted, but she was always available to meet the narcissitic needs of her partner. In return she got validation for her work and some companionship—but at the price of even lower self esteem. As Pat confronted and admitted to this underlying issue we discussed the pattern that linked the food that nourished her and the work that allowed her to avoid her personal pain. Clearly a part of Pat's pattern was the repetitive relationships with men who were never there for her when things got down to the nitty gritty. It paralleled the relationship she had had with her father. She had been the favorite of his four children but felt she never could do enough to satisfy him. And there was always something or someone more important to him than she was when, as a child, she felt particularly needy.

Pat committed herself to avoiding a new relationship until she could learn who she really was and become able to know and assertively ask for what she needed from the people in her life. It was hard, but she told Michael that she felt she deserved more than their ongoing affair. Although she cared very much for Michael she didn't want him to call her anymore.

Their paths did not cross for a year. During that time Pat did some good growth work and came to know and begin to accept herself, warts and all. Being assertive in situations where people she cared about might "go away" was her most difficult obstacle, especially when she found herself around a man she felt powerfully attracted to. When she recognized this powerful attraction as a signal that a potentially addictive, unhealthy relationship was in the wind, she smiled, observed her emotions and moved on.

One day her secretary buzzed her with a call from Michael. A part of Pat knew she should say she could not take the call, but she wanted to see what it felt like to talk to him. Perhaps she was recovered enough to handle herself well. She was glad to hear his voice. She felt that old excitement. A national mental retardation conference was coming up and Michael was wondering if Pat would be there. Yes, she would, she said. Did she have a roommate? Yes, she did. She was staying with her friend, Gwen, and the two women were looking forward to spending some quality time together. When Michael assured Pat he was looking forward to seeing her again, she had to acknowledge a rapid heartbeat.

Pat went to the meeting thinking mostly about what it would

be like to see Michael again. She was talking with a conference participant when she looked up and saw him with a
group of their mutual friends. He smiled warmly–she had
forgotten how much she liked his smile–and they exchanged
a hug. Pat was asked to join "the guys" for dinner and she
linked arms with Michael and another of her friends.

It felt like the emotional void
of past relationships.

The dinner was lively and filled with memories. Pat watched
Michael drink a lot of wine. The rest of the group went to
listen to some jazz and she found herself sitting next to
Michael. He squeezed the hand she offered him, and although he didn't say anything she knew he wanted her to
come back to the hotel room with him. She watched him
drink some more and became aware of the distance between
them. It felt like the emotional void of past relationships. She
was scared. But when they returned to the hotel she told him
that the sexual and needy part of her wanted to spend the
night with him but she thought there had been too much
drinking for an intimate evening. Michael admitted he was
too tired for anything but talk tonight but in the morning...his
voice trailed off. Pat said goodnight and watched Michael
accept it somewhat nonchalantly. He said, "See you tomor-
row." Pat went to her own room, feeling lonely but content
that she had not given another part of herself away.

The next day at the conference went well. As they worked
together Pat continued to enjoy Michael's company, his
bright mind and decisive style. She could also see how much
she had grown in the past year, and that Michael was much
the same as he'd been when they last parted. He asked her to
go to dinner. She accepted. He didn't drink. They talked.

She enthusiastically described her professional work and
carefully described her personal growth work. He told her

how much he had missed her, how much he enjoyed her company, and how much he wanted to continue to see her at the future meetings and conferences where their paths would cross. He told her that although he still was not happy in his marriage he wasn't miserable, and that he and his wife pretty much led their own lives. It was "okay" and he knew he would not end it. He said he did not have another relationship and had no intention to. For what it was worth to her, he would be monogamous, in his own way, while they continued to see one another periodically. Pat smiled as she heard his words. It was a bit like being in a movie. Still, she wanted to believe him. She had been celibate for more than a year and she longed to be held, to make love and to wake up with someone there in the morning.

Suddenly Pat fantasized a way she could justify a relationship with Michael that might be acceptable. It would be like the movie, "Same Time Next Year"–no expectations, no commitments–just being there for one another when they were together. She left Gwen a message that she wouldn't be back until early in the morning and spent the night with Michael. She enjoyed it.

Pat did not enjoy returning to her own hotel room the next morning, hoping no one would see her disheveled appearance. She also felt guilty and ashamed. However, in a short time, she justified her actions in her own mind, then reinforced them as she told Gwen where she was coming from. Pat had known Gwen for a long time; Gwen would unconditionally accept her actions, no matter what she had done. Pat spent more time during the conference with Michael, and less with Gwen.

In the course of the remaining three days Pat practiced some assertiveness with Michael. She told him she was no longer willing to pretend that she wasn't spending time with him by going to the meetings separately. Michael didn't make his usual move to take off early each morning. Instead of their former pattern of falling together later in the evening Pat asked for a commitment as to when they might connect later in the day. She got it. Still, the fear of losing him reared its ugly head and she observed herself making other less assertive choices that revealed that her old habits and needs were still active. She was still compromising her new level of self-esteem.

Michael was a logical person. It was one of the traits that made him so successful in his professional and volunteer work. He had an ability to make decisions when they needed to be made. It was one of the reasons Pat admired him. However, his logical style didn't fit with her needs in their relationship. She was the one who reached for his hand, and she could hardly describe his love making as seductive. She was willing to be content with Michael lying against her at night. Although they talked about one another's children and their work and what was going on in the world, on another level the conversation was superficial. Pat avoided asking Michael about his wife. She became more aware of the distance between them, even in their brief periods of intimacy.

When the conference ended Pat realized she would not see or hear from Michael for six months. A regional conference was coming up before then but that would be a demanding time at work and Pat probably would not be able to get way. She realized she did not have the nerve to ask Michael to call or write. She hoped he would. Then she put him and the relationship out of her mind.

Pat and I met for lunch five days before the conference where she and Michael would again cross paths. She had not spoken to him since their last meeting. Then, two days earlier, during a conference call with Michael and several others, he said he was looking forward to seeing her. Gwen had also called and said she had seen Michael at the regional conference with an attractive woman whom Gwen did not recognize. Michael introduced her to Gwen as his wife. It was the first time Michael's wife had traveled with him in years, but this meeting was being held in the town where they had both grown up so they had made this trip together. Pat was glad she hadn't gone.

I asked Pat what she wanted to do about seeing Michael at the annual foundation meeting. She said she wanted to continue their relationship even though she knew it was not in her best interest. She still had no special person in her life and, once again, wanted to be held and loved and taken care of for a few days. As she told me this I saw the sadness in her eyes, the yearning to belong. I became aware of my own struggle to resolve the dilemma of sometimes knowing what I need to do in my heart and not wanting to acknowledge it in my head–a switch from my usual pattern of knowing what I need to do in my head and not being able to make it fit in my heart. Pat grasped my hand and she asked my advice. I told her this time she was on her own and asked her what she thought she deserved. Pat cried softly. She had already told her therapist of her upcoming meeting. Her therapist reminded Pat that once again she was putting herself in the company of a man who wasn't available to her. Pat agreed that any time she made a decision that didn't give her the best she deserved she was compromising her self-esteem, no matter how much she could justify it in her head.

Pat's therapist also did the most loving thing she could do. She told Pat she hoped she could assert to Michael her need to give herself the opportunity to do what would be best for her in the long run. Her therapist added that if Pat did choose to stay with Michael at the foundation meeting a therapy session would be available when Pat returned.

Both Pat and I know that every time we take a step sideways or backwards we prolong our self actualization. Damn, it's such a struggle! Forty or more years of yearning to "belong" don't disappear with two or three or five or sometimes eight years of good personal work. I remember a workshop given by Earnie Larsen, author of <u>Stage II Relationships</u>. A woman in the audience asked Earnie how long it would take for her to get over her yearning for the old self defeating behaviors that had made her life so unmanageable. Earnie asked her how long she'd practiced her "disease". "Twenty," the woman replied. "How long have you been in recovery?," Earnie asked. "Six years," the woman replied as she sighed. We all knew the answer–up to 14 years.

Like Pat, we all struggle with lifetime change. With our old habits beckoning at every turn, new habits don't hang on as steadfastly as we wish they would. That is why, like Pat, we all need a support network to back up our lifestyle changes. Close friends, a good counselor, mental, physical and nutritional health, and groups to support our growth give us the pats on the back we deserve–and the warnings we may not be willing to acknowledge.

Did Pat spend the night with Michael? What would you have done?

BITES
RECIPES
WE'VE SHARED

BY RONDA GATES

TABLE OF CONTENTS

SOUPS AND SAUCES

MAIN DISHES

ON THE SIDE

SWEET TREATS

v

BITES
(we've shared)

When I first sent a draft of this section of the book to an agent, her comment was that some of the recipes "were not sophisticated enough" and there was "nothing new here." She reminded me that there are lots of low fat cookbooks out so why add this section to Nutrition Nuggets. The point is that these marketing strategists believe books about food sell when:

    1. they're written by a famous person, or
    2. they're illustrated with beautiful photographs, or
    3. the recipes read like they'd taste wonderful.

What I would like you to do is trust me. This cookbook section is a collection of recipes that are more in keeping with what I call a Lowfat Lifestyle® On The Go. The recipes come from people like you and me, not technically educated home economists or gourmet cooks. Many were developed by students of my weight management classes and I have acknowledged their contributions. Others have been developed with a focus toward a more gourmet presentation and company tastes. Some are not as low in fat as you may believe they need to be–they are, however, much lower in fat than the traditional way of preparing these dishes.

During a Lifestyles weight management course I take the class on a supermarket excursion. After the class affirms their new knowledge, we retreat to my home where I prepare a four-dish company meal from scratch. I get it on the table in less than ten minutes. Despite all their class learnings about low fat quick cooking, these students are stunned at how tasty and attractive the dishes are even though it took little or no work to prepare them. This experience gives them the courage to be creative in their own kitchens. You will find some of these quick-to-fix recipes that I developed (in order to practice what I preach) in this section.

All these recipes have been taste-tested many times. With the exception of recipes with less than 1 gram of fat per serving or single ingredient foods they were analyzed by N-Square Computing's NUTRITIONIST III diet analysis program. In those cases I have listed calories per serving, grams of fat per serving, and percent fat of the food. There are also hints for managing your kitchen and your eating patterns.

Enjoy!

GETTING STARTED
COOKING CONVERSIONS

The opportunity to change your eating habits may find you scurrying to old cookbooks to modify favorite recipes and to new cookbooks looking for recipes that conform to goals for a balanced and varied diet that is low in fat, low in sugar, and high in fiber. You will also be checking resources that list amounts of foods in recipes and products in a variety of measurements. Here is an equivalency list that might make translate of these terms to measurements you understand:

3 tsps	1 tablespoon
4 tablespoons	1/4 cup
5 1/3 tablespoons	1/3 cup
8 tablespoons	1/2 cup
10 2/3 tablespoons	2/3 cup
12 tablespoons	3/4 cup
16 tablespoons	1 cup
1 cup	1/2 pint (8 fl. oz.)
2 cups	1 pint (16 fl. oz.)
4 cups	1 quart (32 fl. oz.)
2 pints	1 quart (32 fl. oz.)
4 quarts (liquid)	1 gallon (128 fl. oz.)
8 quarts (dry)	1 peck
4 pecks (dry)	1 bushel
1 tablespoon	5 milliliters
1 cup	236.5 milliliters
1 pint	473 milliliters
1 quart	946 milliliters (about 1 liter)
1 gallon	3.79 liters
1 peck	7.57 liters
1 bushel	30.28 liters
1 ounce	28.35 grams
1 pound	454 grams (approximately)
2 1/20 pounds	1 kilogram
1.06 quarts	1 liter

And, here are some COOKING EQUIVALENTS for dry measures that should also help you in and out of the kitchen.

3 tablespoons flour	1 ounce
3 1/2 to 4 cups flour	1 pound
2 cups granulated sugar	1 pound
2 1/4 cups packed brown sugar	1 pound
4 cups confectioners' sugar(approx.)	1 pound
2 tablespoons butter	1 ounce
2 cups uncooked rice	1 pound
2 3/8 cups raisins	1 pound
1 cup nutmeats	1/4 pound
4 medium potatoes	1 pound
4 cups sliced medium apples	1 1/2 pounds
1 square unsweetened chocolate	1 ounce
4 ounces American cheese	1 cup shredded
8 egg whites	1 cup
8 egg yolks	3/4 cup
28 saltine crackers	1 cup fine crumbs
1 slice bread	1/4 cup fine crumbs
7 ounces spaghetti	4 cups cooked
2 cups rice	4 cups cooked
1 medium onion	1/2 cup chopped
1 medium lemon	3 tablespoons juice
1 medium orange	1/3 cup juice
10 tablespoons flour	100 grams
7 tablespoons granulated sugar	100 grams
10 tablespoons brown sugar	100 grams
3/4 cup confectioners' sugar	100 grams
7 tablespoons butter	100 grams
5/8 cup less 1 tablespoons raisins	100 grams

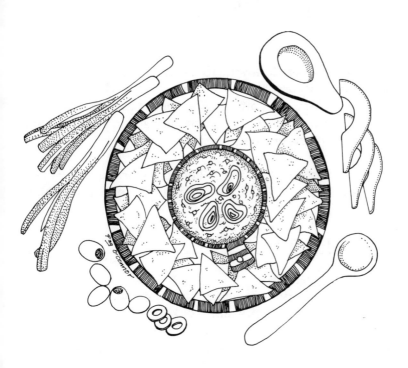

NIBBLES AND BITES

When you decide to eat lower-in-fat you may discover benefits that go beyond the lower body fat image you desire. It is well known that decisions that affect your well being enhance self esteem. My experience is that enhanced creativity goes hand in hand with feeling good about myself. I have put that creativity to work for me in the kitchen. Discovering low fat ways to snack has become a creative and satisfying hobby for me. I am one of those people willing to eat whatever is easily available so I still take advantage of the abundant fresh fruits and vegetables that are available year around in most supermarkets. But, I have also taken the risk of experimenting in my kitchen, and the result is a few recipes that are good substitutes for the higher in fat snack foods you find on your grocer's shelves. Here are a few of them:

Tortillas are a terrific low fat food that can be made into chips or be the basis for other lowfat snack foods or dishes. For non fat tortilla chips use corn tortillas–the more coarse the better (In the Pacific Northwest many stores carry El Ranchito brand which are the best I've tried).

P. S. Although most people believe corn tortillas have no fat they are, in fact, 12% fat. The fat comes from the natural oil in corn.

LOW FAT TORTILLA CHIPS

<u>Microwave version</u>
Pass the corn tortilla under running water and lay it flat in a microwave. You can probably cook three at a time, but they should not be stacked. "Nuke" on high setting for about a minute and a half for each tortilla. (Ovens vary in wattage so you'll have to experiment). If you flip them mid-cooking they will be more crisp.

<u>Oven Version</u>
Pass the corn tortilla under running water and lay it flat in your oven. Lay a glass dish on top of them to assure they stay flat. Bake at about 400 o until crisp. Watch this process the first few times so you can adjust the temperature and assure the tortillas don't burn.

After cooking you can leave the crisped tortillas whole and stack them vertically in a cloth lined basket or break them into pieces for dipping.

One tortilla: 67 calories, 1 gm fat, 12% fat.

NON FAT BEAN DIP

Commercial bean dip is filled with fat, usually saturated and often lard. You can make your own non fat bean dip by blending:

1 can of pinto beans, drained
Salsa to taste

Believe it or not, that's all.

One 8 oz. cup: 399.7 calories, 2.83 gm fat, 6% fat.

FRESH TOMATO SALSA

1 clove garlic, minced
1/4 cup chopped parsley
1/3 cup chopped cilantro
1 large onion
4 tomatoes, coarsely chopped
1 pickled jalapeno
3 Tbs. red wine vinegar
1 Tbs. olive oil
2 dashes Tabasco
Salt and pepper to taste

Mix together all ingredients. Makes about 4 cups.

150 calories, 4.9 gm fat, 18% fat.
(Omit the olive oil and it is virtually fat free.)

LOWFAT NACHOS

My son would live on nachos if he could so we experimented with a variety of ways to combine chips, cheese, beans, salsa and guacamole until we came up with this!

Make the corn tortilla chipss described on page 6. Break them into pieces and put them in a glass dish that has been sprayed with non stick vegetable spray. If you like, cover them with the bean dip above. Grate part skim mozarella cheese and part skim cheddar cheese (Weight Watchers and Kraft make a lower in fat brand) over the chips. Bake or microwave until the cheese melts. Top with salsa (most brands are non fat) and, if desired, with Zesty Avocado Dressing (see Salads and Salad Dressing section) that has been thickened with Yogurt Cheese (also in Salads and Salad Dresssing section). If desired, top with non fat plain yogurt.

• If you've never eaten very low fat foods, experiment with low fat yogurt or other varieties of cheeses for in-between small steps to reach your ultimate low fat goal.

1 oz. serving: 62 calories, 1.3 gm fat 19% fat

TORTILLA STACKS

Three Crisped Corn Tortillas.
2 Slices of Weight Watchers Cheese.
Alternate tortillas and cheese in a stack.
Heat in a microwave until the cheese has melted.
Eat as is or cut into triangles (this is a little messy) and enjoy.

• You can also dip these triangled "sandwich snacks" in salsa for a finger lickin' good nacho!

280 calories, 7 gm fat and is 23% fat.

SALMON BALL

This salmon ball recipe is a modification of a traditional recipe that was served at parties for years. Now that low fat cream cheese products are available, the fat level can be decreased slightly. Remember, I said *slightly*. This is such a good hors d'oeuvre that you may be tempted to eat more than you want or need. If you use salmon canned in oil, be sure to rinse it before you prepare this dish.

1 6 oz. can red salmon
1 8 oz. low fat cream cheese product, softened
1 Tbs. lemon juice
2 tsp. grated onion (use green onion and tops chopped)
1 tsp. prepared white horseradish
1 tsp. salt
1/4 tsp. Liquid Smoke
3 tbs. snipped parsley, chopped.

Drain and flake salmon removing skin and bones. Combine the remaining ingredients–except parsley–and mix thoroughly. Chill several hours. Shape salmon mixture into a ball and roll in parsley. Chill well. Serve with low fat crackers (melba is a good choice) or on thin rye bread.

• If you can't get Weight Watchers low fat cream cheese, mix whipped cream cheese (70% fat as opposed to regular cream cheese which is 90% fat) with some Yogurt Cheese

• Substitute crab or imitation crab for the salmon for a lower in fat dish.

16 servings
27.4 calories, 1.1 gm fat, 28% fat

EGGPLANT CAPONATA

This is an excellent hors d'oeuvre or first course, served on toasted french bread.

1 eggplant, sliced lengthwise
1 tsp. salt
1/2 cup chicken broth
2 stalks celery, diced
1/3 cup red onion, diced
1 tsp. capers
4 Roma tomatoes, diced
3 Tbs. tomato paste
1 tsp. sugar
2 Tbs. olive oil
3 Tbs. Balsamic vinegar
1 1/2 Tbs. fresh basil and parsley, chopped
1/2 Tbs. garlic, finely chopped.

Using a non-stick pan, saute eggplant in chicken stock. Saute diced onion and celery in remaining stock until softened. Transfer to a bowl with eggplant. Add remaining ingredients and season to taste with salt and pepper. Keeps up to 2 weeks in the refrigerator. Serve at room temperature and re-season after storing for a while.

•One teaspoon of dried herbs is equivilent to 3 teaspoons of fresh herbs.

12 servings
64 calories, 2.3 gm fat, 31% fat.

VEGETABLE CRISPS

1/2 inch slices of zucchini, sliced onion, cauliflower or
      broccoli flowerets or any other vegetable suitable for
      snacking
Vegetable cooking spray
2 Tbs. reduced-calorie mayonnaise
2 Tbs. minced green onions
1 Tbs. dijon or other seasoned mustard
Marjoram and/or thyme seasoning
3/4 cup soft whole wheat or oat bran bread crumbs
1/2 tsp. paprika
1 Tbs. melted margarine

Place vegetables on a baking sheet coated with cooking
spray. Combine mayonnaise and next three ingredients; stir
well. Spread 1/2 tsp. of mayonnaise mixture over each
vegetable. Combine remaining ingredients; stir well. Sprinkle
evenly over zucchini, turning to turning to coat well. Bake at
450°for 5 minutes or until bread crumbs are browned. Serve
warm.

Yield about 2 dozen appetizers with less than one gram fat
each.

* Non fat plain yogurt is a satisfying substitute for reduced-
calorie mayonnaise in dishes that have seasonings addded

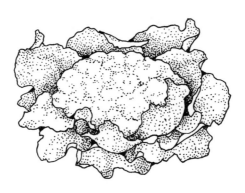

Hang in there with me on this one—it is hard to believe this will work until you try it—and, you will have to do some trial and error experimenting to get the timing and consistency appropriate to your microwave down pat.

CHEESE MELT

Cut a 1/4 inch slice of part skim mozzarella cheese and put it on a plate that is suitable for microwaving. Using a high setting, melt the cheese then CONTINUE to heat it until it congeals again and becomes chewy looking. You can roll it in balls for a delicious snack or spread it on a crisp cracker like Ry Crisp or Wasa bread. (You'll also be able to use a paper towel to blot additional oil from the cheese after cooking.)

Part skim mozarella cheese is 56% fat

HIGH FAT CHEESES
Brie
Muenster
Cheddar
American
Swiss

LOWFAT CHEESES (50% or less)
Part skim mozarella
Lappi
Farmer's
Weight Watchers brand

Use flank steak , one of the leaner cuts of beef, for making your own beef jerky. Remember, beef jerky is salty and is not suitable for people at high risk for cardiac disease.

BEEF JERKY

1 1/2 lbs. flank steak
1 tsp. MSG
1 tsp. liquid smoke
1 tsp. onion powder
1/3 tsp. pepper
1/4 cup Worcestershire
1/3 tsp. garlic powder
1/4 cup soy sauce.

Partially freeze the flank steak and slice into long very thin 1/4" slices, making sure to remove all fat. Marinate for a minimum 24 hours (or longer). Drain in a colander and place on a broiler pan rack. Bake at 150° with the oven door ajar overnight or for ten hours.

24 servings
58.5 calories, 1.76 gm fat, 28% fat.

One of my favorite appetizers continues to be variations of the Quiche Qubes recipe found in <u>Lowfat Lifestyle</u>. Here is an even lower in fat version of the original and some suggestions on how to make it more versatile.

QUICHE QUBES AGAIN

3/4 cup grated part-skim mozzarella cheese
3/4 cup grated Kraft reduced calorie cheddar cheese
1 teaspoon Italian seasoning
2 ounces diced turkey ham
1 egg + 2 egg whites
1 cup non fat skim milk

Use a 1 quart baking dish sprayed with non-stick cooking spray. Sprinkle grated cheeses, seasoning and turkey ham into the dish and stir gently to mix.

Beat together egg, egg whites and milk and pour over the mixture in the pan, stirring until everything is well mixed. Bake at 350° for 45 minutes or until cheese is firmly set. Serve hot or cold.

Makes 24 cubes

20 calories, 1.1 gram fat, 50% fat

VARIATIONS
Add thinly sliced red or green peppers
Add thinly sliced or grated onion
Add thinly sliced mushrooms
Substitute shrimp for the turkey ham
Add thinly sliced zucchini that has been stir fried in broth
Add thawed and well drained chopped spinach
        (previously frozen!)
Substitute reduced calorie swiss cheese for the cheddar
        cheese.

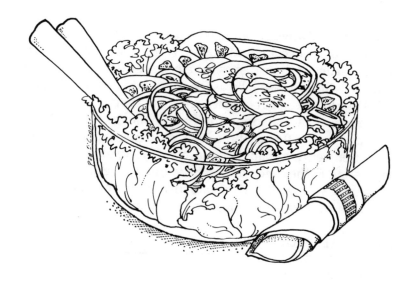

SALADS
and
SALAD DRESSINGS

Salads are the "way to go" to increase complex carbohydrates and provide the binding fiber that is so important to a healthy diet. Fresh fruits and vegetables are considered fat free and the more of them you eat the lower in fat your total diet will be. I encourage you to keep leafy lettuce and spinach in your refrigerator along with a variety of non fat salad dressings and the trimmings (green onions, 3 bean salad, parmesan cheese, tomatoes, celery, sliced carrots, water chestnuts, assorted peppers, etc.) to be able to "throw together" a salad on a moments notice. Beyond the green varieties that are easy to create on your own, here are a few that take a little more preparation (but they are worth it). The salad dressings follow!

Jello recipes always get a mixed reaction from my audiences because Jello is so high in sugar. Well, now that there are sugar-free Jellos these dishes have been re-added to the diets of those willing to use Jello as food for more than healing the sick. I like Jello recipes because they are so adaptable. With one basic recipe I have an opportunity to challenge my creativity by changing the flavor of the Jello, changing the ingredients or, better yet, by changing the mold. If your mold has a depression in the center add extra yogurt or fresh fruit there. Serve molds on an attractive plate surrounded by small leaves and fresh fruit for a more festive presentation.

TROPICAL VEGETABLE SALAD

1 3 oz. package of lemon or orange Jello
1 small can pineapple chunks, in own juice, drained
1/2 cup grated carrots
1/2 cup chopped celery.

Dissolve Jello as directed in 1/2 cup hot water. Mix the juice from the drained pineapple with enough water to make 1 1/2 cups, and add to the Jello water. Add the pineapple, carrots and celery. Refrigerate until molded.

Serves 6.
19.6 calories/serving, 45 gm fat, 3% fat.

QUICK TO FIX FRUIT SALAD

For quick-to-fix salads, buy bags of frozen fruit at a wholesale or discount market. Make a dressing with vanilla flavored yogurt cheese.

•This also makes a terrific dessert.

This recipe was brought to class by Judy Wolson, a student in my first Minnesota Lifestyles® class. When Judy first modified this recipe the variety of non-fat yogurts available today were unknown. I've left the recipe as it came to me, calling for Lean or Lite sour cream. After your tastes change and you want still lower in fat foods try one of the non-fat products instead of the sour cream. You can also substitute fresh fruit for canned fruit in the summertime.

BLUEBERRY JELLO MOLD

1 pkg. sugar free raspberry Jello
1 pkg. sugar free strawberry Jello
2 cups boiling water
1 can water packed blueberries (drained) (2 cups)
1/2 pint Lean sour cream.

Mix gelatin with hot water. Cool until partially set, then whip gelatin and fold in blueberries then sour cream. Pour into mold and chill until set.

8 servings

<u>With non fat yogurt</u>
37.8 calories/serving
.18 gm of fat
4% fat

<u>With not lean sour cream</u>
83.5 calories/serving
6.16 gm of fat
64% fat

ORIENTAL CHICKEN SALAD

1 whole chicken breast, boned and skinned before cooking in
microwave or oven without added fat or oil
3 oz snow peas cooked slightly and sliced lengthwise
4 black peppercorns
1 celery rib, thinly sliced
4 mushrooms, thinly sliced
1/4 cup scallions, thinly sliced

Moisten with drained non fat yogurt thinned with rice
vinegar. Add a touch of soy sauce if desired.

2-3 servings
118 calories, 2.23 grams of fat, 17% fat

•Try a combination of chunk chicken, cantalope, strawberries and grapes in a salad. You will love it.

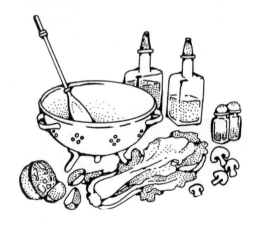

CHICKEN AND SPINACH SALAD

2 whole medium chicken breasts, skinned and boned
4 cups spinach
1 sweet red pepper, cut into strips
1 hot yellow chili pepper, seeded and chopped
Nonfat Weight Watchers Salad Dressing
*Optional for cold dish: 1/4 cup nonfat yogurt

Cut chicken into thin strips. Marinate in salad dressing, covered, in the refrigerator. Toss together spinach and peppers. Drain chicken; reserve marinade. Stir-fry chicken in non-stick skillet until tender. Add reserved marinade to skillet and cook over high heat one minute. Remove from heat. Pour over spinach, toss one minute or until spinach slightly wilts. Add chicken.

4 servings

*This can also be prepared as a cold salad by adding the stir-fried chicken to the spinach Toss with the reserved salad dressing mixed with two Tbs. of nonfat yogurt.

167 calories, 3.37 grams of fat, 19% fat

•Sweet yellow or green bell peppers are suitable substitutes if you have difficulty finding the bright red sweet peppers that color lots of low fat recipes.

IMITATION CRAB SALAD

The sweet cherry tomatoes are the secret ingredient in this salad.

1/2 pound imitation crab meat
1 cup chopped celery
1/2 cup chopped green onions
1 small can sliced water chestnuts
1/2 basket ripe cherry tomatoes
1/2 cup low fat ranch salad dressing
(I use packaged mix prepared with 1/2 reduced calorie mayonnaise and 1/2 non fat yogurt)

Mix all the ingredients EXCEPT the tomatoes.
Just before serving slice the tomatoes in half and add to the salad.

4 servings
154 calories, 9 grams of fat, 23% fat

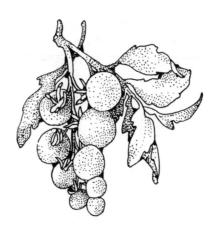

COUSCOUS SALAD

(You have to make this ahead and chill it—but that makes it a meal in 5 minutes!)

1 package of frozen cut green beans
      (or mixed beans or mixed vegetables)
1 1/3 cup ready-to-cook couscous
6 oz. turkey pastrami
1/2 cup low fat Italian salad dressing
      (or a non-fat Italian)
Optional: Weight Watchers packaged Chicken Broth or
      Pritikin canned Chicken Broth

Cook vegetables according to package directions. Drain well. Meanwhile, place couscous in a large mixing bowl. Pour 1 1/3 cup boiling water over couscous. Let stand 5 minutes. Cut the turkey pastrami into wedges. Stir pastrami, cooked beans and dressing into couscous. Mix well. Cover and chill for 3 hours or more. Serve on lettuce leaves as is, or mixed into a variety of torn lettuce as a tossed salad.

175 calories, 4.8 grams of fat, 24% fat (with low fat dressing)

CORN, CILANTRO AND RED PEPPER SALAD

2 16 oz. cans corn
1 large red bell pepper, diced
1 bunch chopped cilantro

Combine all ingredients and enjoy!

Serves 4–6 people.
64 calories, less than 1 gram of fat, 10% fat

This salad is wonderful and incredibly easy!

MIXED VEGETABLE SALAD

Cut into small pieces:
> cauliflower
> broccoli
> carrots
> celery
> mushrooms
> cherry tomatoes
> water chestnuts

Marinate in 3 Tablespoons of non fat Italian dressing for at least 8 hours before serving.

Negligable calories

• Use frozen vegetables in salads to given them a crispy texture. To quick cool a can of food you are going to use right away, open the can and put it in the freezer section for 20 minutes.

• Lettuce wedges are much faster to prepare than a tossed salad and they go well with casseroles, stews, and soups

• Although it is bulky to store, a salad cripser that whirls the moisture out of washed salads will save you lots of time when you are cutting and storing greens for future use.

COTTAGE CHEESE SALAD

1 cup low fat cottage cheese
1/4 cup cucumber peeled, sliced and diced
1/4 cup celery, thinly sliced
4 thin slices red onion
4 red radishes, thinly sliced
1 Tbs. fresh dill, chopped

Mix together and chill. Add shrimp or water packed tuna for a main course.

• Keep a can of water packed tuna in your refrigerator. It adds chill to salads quickly.

4 servings
102 calories, 1.5 grams of fat, 13% fat

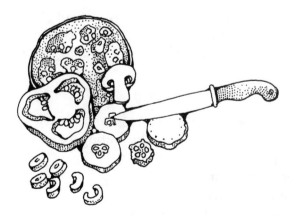

ABOUT YOGURT CHEESE

Although you may have come across this recipe in other cookbooks I have added it here because it has been the most versatile use of yogurt I have found. Open my refrigerator and you will find at least two cartons of yogurt being drained for use in another way. Yogurt cheese can be used as a base for sauces, salad dressings, desserts and dessert toppings.

YOGURT CHEESE

Line a funnel with cheesecloth or use a coffee filter. Spoon yogurt into the lined funnel or filter. Support it in a bowl and drain it overnight in your refrigerator. In the morning the whey (the liquid part of the yogurt) will have separated out and you will have a non fat cream cheese textured food that is wonderful as a base for salads, sauces, condiments and dessert toppings. Use yogurt cheese to cut the fat in a variety of recipes. Try this with a variety of brands of yogurt. Some brands are sweet and some are sour. You may find you prefer one for desserts, and another for condiments and sauces!!
•Mix yogurt cheese with a non fat salad dressing for creamy non fat salad toppings.
•Mix yogurt cheese with a variety of mustards for sandwiches.
• Remember there is regular yogurt (about 25% fat) , lowfat yogurt (15% fat) and non-fat yogurt (no fat). Choose according to the amount of fat you *don't* want in your diet.

•Coffee filters are also useful to:
absorb drips from popsicles by putting the stick through the center of the filter
separate your non-stick pans
separate your dishes
hold tacos and other finger foods

CREAMY SALAD DRESSING

(measurements approximate–adjust to taste)
2 1/2 cups of non fat plain yogurt
1/3 cup frozen apple juice concentrate
1/4 cup vinegar
1/4 cup parmesan cheese
2 Tbs. olive oil
1/4 cup juice from canned beets (optional)
3 Tbs. dried chopped onions
1 Tbs. Italian seasoning
1/2 tsp. garlic powder
1/2 envelope unflavored gelatin
1/4 cup water.

Soften the gelatin in a small amount of cold water. Add 1/4 cup of boiling water to dissolve. Add to other ingredients in the blender, blend, chill and stir. Store in the refrigerator.

Makes 3 cups
41.5 calories, 1.5 grams of fat, 30% fat per tablespoon

RANCH YOGURT DRESSING OR DIP
Kaye Van Valkenburg

2 cups plain non-fat yogurt
1 1/2 tsp. dill weed
1 1/4 tsp. onion powder
1 tsp. garlic powder
1 tsp. dried chives
1/4 tsp. dried basil
pinch ground white pepper
salt as desired
2 Tbs. powdered non-fat milk
2 tsp. white vinegar

Mix all ingredients thoroughly. For best flavor, make several hours before needed. Keeps well in refrigerator.
Each tablespoon of dip has about 11 calories.

There are so many delicious nonfat salad dressings on the market and so many seasoning packets available that can be mixed with non-fat yogurt and/or light mayonnaise that I no longer have any occasion to concoct my own dressings. My favorite continues to be one I adopted from a recipe originally published by Carla Mulligan and Eve Lowry but which is not in their recommended cookbook <u>Lean Life Cuisine</u>.

ZESTY AVOCADO DRESSING

1 ripe avocado
2/3 cup non-fat buttermilk
1/3 cup lowfat cottage cheese (1% now available)
1 tsp. Worchestershire sauce
1/8 tsp. garlic powder
1/8 tsp. salt
Dash cayenne pepper

Put all ingredients in a blender and blend until smooth. Thicken, if desired, with yogurt cheese.

40 calories, 1.3 grams of fat, 40% fat per tablespoon

• This dressing can also be used, when blended with yogurt cheese, (see page 24) as a lowfat guacamole dip or as a topping for Mexican dishes.

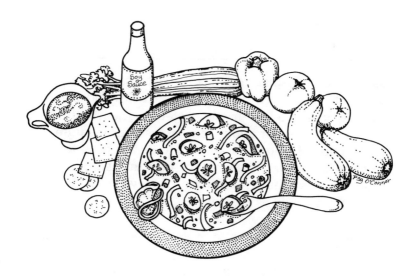

SOUPS AND SAUCES

There are only a few of these but I have added them because whenever I serve them they are a hit. They rarely require fat, smell wonderful while they cook and served with a salad and hot bread make a hearty meal.

When you cook soups prepare double portions, cool what you don't use and freeze the leftovers in one-meal containers. Remove individual servings from the freezer in the morning and reheat them in your oven or microwave just before dinner.

Don't overlook packaged soup mixes in your grocery stores, gourmet cooking stores or delicatessens. Even the more expensive soup mixes sell for under $5 a package and make six to eight servings. With bread and a tossed salad you have a hearty gourmet meal for less than $1.00 per person.

VEGETABLE STOCK

Using water or a small amount of olive oil, saute onion, garlic and herbs in a stock pot. Add vegetables and begin the cooking process by stir-frying or stewing them with a small amount of water for about 15 minutes over medium heat. Add 8 cups of water (for about 7 to 8 cups of vegetables). Bring to a boil and then reduce heat and simmer for 45 minutes. Pour the stock through a sieve pressing out as much of the liquid as possible.

Makes 6 cups.

Suggested vegetables: Carrots, onions, leek greens, celery stalks and leaves, squash, potatoes, potato parings, lettuce and parsley leaves. Season with thyme, bay leaf, sage, garlic, salt and/or pepper.

18% fat

CHICKEN STOCK

For the best chicken stock, the less fleshy chicken parts–backs, necks and wings–make the best soup. Add leftover vegetables to make the stock more hearty but don't use too much of one vegetable–it will overpower the chicken flavor. Avoid celery–it adds a bitter, salty flavor.

Place your ingredients in a stock pot. Cover with cold water and simmer 4 hours.
Makes up to 8 cups.

• Suggested vegetables for chicken broth include: Mushroom stems, tomatoes, carrots, parsley stems, celery and thyme branches. In addition, add peppercorns, salt, and a bay leaf or two.

30% fat

QUICK TOMATO SAUCE

2 28 oz. cans of Italian tomatoes, coarsely chopped
1 large onion, finely diced
3 Tbs. chopped garlic
1/2 cup tomato paste
1 tsp. each oregano, basil and thyme
1 Tbs. olive oil

Heat olive oil in a heavy non-aluminum pan. Add onions
and cook until soft. Add garlic. Cook for 2 minutes and add
the rest of the ingredients. Let simmer for 15 minutes or so.
Season to taste with salt and pepper.

30% fat with olive oil
Negligible fat without olive oil

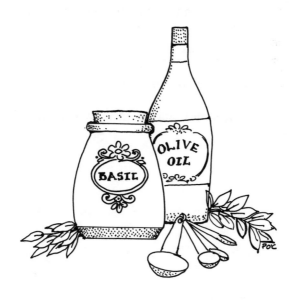

BEEF VEGETABLE SOUP
Barb Garrett, Minneapolis

1 lb. extra lean ground beef
1 tsp. brown bouquet sauce
3 cups water
3 carrots, chopped
2 stalks celery, chopped
1 lg. potato, chopped
2 med. onions
1 can tomato sauce and 1 cup of water or 1 can of V-8 juice.
1 1/2 tsp. salt
1/4 to 1/2 tsp. pepper
1 bay leaf
1/2 tsp. basil
1 14 oz. can of tomatoes
1/3 cup alphabet noodles

Cook hamburger in a non-stick coated skillet. Drain off any fat and blot the meat. Stir in the remaining ingredients. Heat to boiling then simmer until tender. Add a little seasoning salt and Accent, if desired. Add the noodles, tomato sauce and cook until the noodles are tender.

8 servings
179 calories, 5 grams of fat, 26% fat

• The alphabet noodles makes this an enticing dish for children!

CURRIED LENTIL SOUP

1 1/2 cups chicken broth or stock
1/3 cup chopped onion
a garlic clove, minced
1 tsp. finely chopped ginger
1/2 Tbs. curry powder or to taste
1/2 tsp. ground cumin
1/2 cup lentils, picked over and rinsed
1/2 cup chopped, drained canned tomatoes
1 cup firmly packed coarsely chopped spinach leaves,
        washed well
fresh lemon juice to taste

In a large heavy saucepan cook the onion in 3 tablespoons chicken broth, stirring until it is lightly golden. Add the garlic and the ginger and cook the mixture, stirring, for 1 minute. Add the curry powder and cumin, cook for 30 seconds, and add the lentils and 1 1/4 cups water. Bring the liquid to a boil and simmer the mixture, covered , for 25 minutes. Stir in the tomatoes and the spinach and simmer the soup, stirring occasionally, for 2 minutes. Season the soup with the lemon juice and salt and pepper to taste.
3 8-oz.. servings

160 calories, less than 1 gram of fat, 5% fat

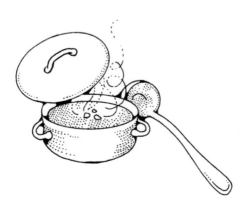

ZUCCHINI SOUP

1 medium chopped onion
2 medium finely chopped zucchini
4 cups tomato juice
1 can de-fatted chicken broth or stock
3 Tbs. lime juice
2 tsps. Worcestershire
1 tsp. salt, pepper & sugar
1/4 - 1/2 tsp. Tabasco
2 Tbs. chopped parsley
Use bay leaf, garlic and/or Italian herbs to taste
Parmesan to decorate

Saute onions in a teflon pan until soft (5 minutes). Stir in zucchini and saute for 2-3 minutes. Add tomato juice, chicken broth, lime juice, Worchestershire, spices, salt, pepper and sugar. Simmer for fifteen minutes. Stir in chopped parsley. After ladling into serving dishes sprinkle top with parmesan cheese.

8 servings
52 calories, less than 1 gram of fat, 14% fat

OPTION: Add extra lean ground beef to the soup for protein.

PUTTANESCA

1/2 cup chicken stock
3 cloves chopped garlic
2 Tbs. capers
1 Tbs. finely chopped anchovies
2 cups tomato sauce
2 tsp. each parsley and basil

Saute garlic in stock for about 15 seconds in very hot pan. Add remaining ingredients, heating thoroughly. Season with salt and pepper. Toss with pasta. Serves 2.

149 calories, 1.5 grams of fat, 10% fat

•Use de-fatted chicken broth as a base for sauces for pastas and stew.

•Thicken soups and stews with low fat cheese products.

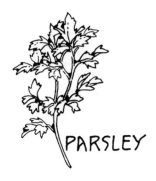

PARSLEY

AND YOU CAN ALSO...

Toss a couple of microwaved until done, cut, red potatoes in a can of heated low fat soup. (Progressosoups are the lowest in fat and salt I have found as this goes to press.) Top it with low fat grated swiss or cheddar cheese.

or

Add a cup of cooked brown rice and 1/2 cup of frozen corn to low in fat chicken broth. Top the "soup" with non fat frozen yogurt. If you make this very thick and want it a more south of the border taste, add some salsa.

or

Saute' strips of lean steak or boneless breast of chicken in spicy V-8. Add leftover wild rice and more V-8 to the desired consistency.

or

Make any gazpacho recipe without the oil called for in the recipe.

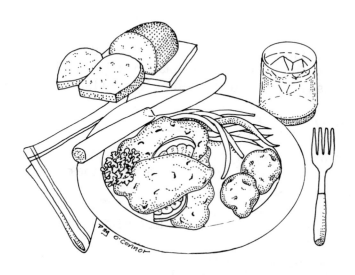

MAIN DISHES

Many of the people who enter my classes believe they will have to give up the recipes that have given them reputations as cooks with a magic touch. Not so! My watchword is MODIFY.

The first key to low fat cooking is to substitute your fancy gourmet cookwear with more efficient non-stick cookwear. You will be able to cut the fat in every main dish recipe you have by half *without* compromising the taste. Practice substituting higher in fat condiments like sour cream and cheese with lower in fat varieties. (See Quick Starts on page 21 of Nutrition Nuggets.)

Remember! Decreasing the fat in a meal by only 100 calories can add up to a one-half pound weight loss in a week. That is two pounds a month or 25 pounds a year. Non-fat recipes are not the goal of lowfat lifestyle cooking–*lower* in fat recipes are the goal.

Later in the class there is a lot of sharing of recipes for chicken, fish, beef and yes, even pork dishes. Here are some that have been favorites.

I put the potato bar in this section because in this form it is a main dish. This is a versatile adaptation of the popular salad bar and is a happy option for feeding large and small groups.

POTATO BAR

Microwave or bake large red or baking potatoes until done. (The cooking time will depend on the size of the potato and method of cooking.)

Prepare an array of toppings and let guests choose from:
> salsa
> shredded low fat cheese
> light cream cheese mixed with yogurt cheese
> parmesan cheese
> light sour cream or plain low fat or non fat yogurt
> home cooked or canned chili
> chopped tomatoes
> chopped onions
> ready to serve hearty soups
> undiluted condensed lowfat soups
> seasoned mustards mixed with yogurt cheese
> steamed broccoli

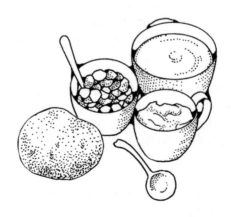

You can also use this same idea to prepare a pasta bar. Prepare two or three different pastas and offer the toppings below.

PASTA BAR

Use any of the suggestions for potatoes (above) or use:
Canned tomato paste mixed with spicy V-8 Juice and Italian seasoning
A mixture of low fat ricotta and Weight Watchers swiss cheese or part skim milk, mozarella cheese and yogurt cheese (page 24).
Mix clams or diced chicken or shrimp in pasta as a condiment.

Notes about pasta
•The oil in pasta recipes prevents the pasta from sticking together and to the pan. If you stir your pasta as you cook and if you use non-stick cookwear you don't need the oil.
•Use at least three quarts of water for eight ounces of pasta. You'll be able to satisfy at least four hearty appetites.
•Recipes apply to any of a variety of pastas currently available (fresh, frozen, dry packaged, vegetable based, preseasoned, curled, straight and shaped).
•Don't add pasta to the pan until the water is boiling vigorously. After adding pasta, begin cooking time when the water returns to a boil. Stir to prevent boiling over.
•Drain pasta immediately after cooking.
•If you're using low fat canned sauces or cheese for pasta you don't have to heat them. Just add them to the hot pasta and the meal will be at serving temperature about the time everything is mixed together.
•If you're topping pasta with regular or part skim milk cheese, melt it in the microwave before adding it to the pasta. The fat in the cheese will rise to the top and can be blotted away with a paper towel. You'll be surprised how much fat you can remove this way!

CHICKEN FAJITAS

One pound skinless-boneless breast of chicken, sliced
One green, red and yellow pepper, sliced
One medium onion, sliced
One package whole wheat tortillas
One head of iceburg lettuce shredded
Chopped tomato or mild salsa
Grated low fat cheese for garnish
Non fat plain yogurt, low fat sour cream or yogurt cheese
    (see page 24) if desired
* One package Fajita Seasoning

Spray a large teflon pan with Pam. Heat the pan to medium hot. Place chicken in pan–not necessary to stir. When you turn the chicken add the sliced vegetables.Don't stir for about five minutes. The steam will cook the vegetables.When finished cooking, stir and mix chicken and vegetables. Season, if you think it's necessary, with Fajita seasoning. Wrap tortillas in baking paper or cheesecloth and warm in a microwave oven or wrap in foil and warm in a 350° oven. Put 1/4-1/2 cup of chicken mixture in tortilla. Cover with lettuce, tomato, and grated cheese. Roll if desired or serve open faced. This serves 6-8 depending on size of tortilla.

*If you want a more seasoned dish, marinate the sliced chicken in the package of Fajita Seasoning according to directions before you cook the chicken.

218 calories, 5 grams of fat, 21% fat

MEXICAN CHICKEN

---

1 medium onion, chopped
1 clove garlic, minced
1 cup V-8 juice
1 Tbs. Mexican seasoning (or use 1 tsp. basil, 1 tsp. oregano,
1 tsp. chili powder)
3 cups of boned, skinned, cooked (without fat) chicken breast
1 small can chopped green chiles
1/2 cup grated low fat cheddar cheese
Two corn tortillas dried until crisp then crushed*

Combine onion, garlic, V-8 juice, and seasonings a in saucepan and simmer for one hour. In a baking dish, layer the
chicken, chili, and cheese. Top with the sauce. Sprinkle top
with crushed tortilla chips. Bake 30 minutes at 350°.

*See page 6 for instructions on how to dry the tortillas).

Despite the long list of ingredients, this turkey tetrazzini
recipe is easy and fast to cook. It's a great way to use leftover

319 calories, 9.6 grams of fat, 28% fat

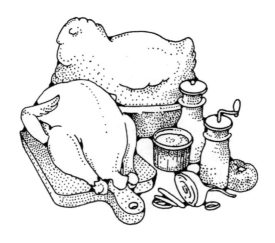

This is a good and easy recipe. Any herbs can be used.

BAKED CHICKEN BREAST
WITH DIJON AND LEMON JUICE

2 chicken breasts, boned and skinned.
1/4 cup lemon juice
2 Tbs. Dijon mustard
1 tsp. each rosemary and thyme.

Spray a glass baking dish with vegetable spray. Sprinkle breasts with lemon juice, brush with Dijon and sprinkle herbs evenly over breasts. Bake in a preheated 350° oven for 35 minutes.

Serves 2.
311 calories, 6.5 grams of fat, 20% fat

•Many super discount markets offer lower prices when you make bulk purchases. Look for boneless, skinless breasts in five pound packages. Before you leave the house in the morning take the amount required for a recipe from the freezer and put it in the refrigerator. It will be thawed when you return home. (Frozen chicken can also be thawed quickly in the microwave for instant use.)

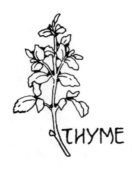

THYME

GAME HENS A L' ORANGE

Game hens have always been one of my favorite choices for special occasion dinners. They are pretty high in fat, compared to other poultry, but you can remove the skin and voila!–you have a low fat company meal. I have often been able to slide a large piece of skin off the hen, cooked it separately, then placed it back on top of the hen when I serve it to satisfy people who prefer a less bare look. For a tasty, well rounded, and colorful dinner, combine this recipe with wild rice and a green vegetable such as broccoli or asparagus sprinkled with Molly McButter.

4 Cornish game hens cut in half
vegetable spray
white pepper
2 lg. onions, quartered
1 6 oz. can frozen orange juice concentrate, thawed
2 cups dry white wine.

Preheat the oven to 350°. Spray the vegetable coating on your hands and rub the game hens so that it will hold the white pepper you sprinkle on top.Place the halves in a shallow roasting pan, cut side down on onion quarters. Put them in the preheated oven for 15 minutes. Combine the orange juice concentrate and white wine, then pour it over the hens. Continue to cook another 45 minutes, basting every 5-10 minutes.Remove from oven and place on serving platter or individual plates. Pour the sauce over the hens before serving.

8 servings
447 calories, 6.4 grams of fat, 13% fat

• This recipe is also delicious using boneless breast of chicken.
•For my friends who avoid alcohol–use a seltzer water instead of wine.
•Try different juices for different tastes.

CROCK POT CHICKEN
Bev Holtzer (Kansas City)

3-4 lbs. chicken (skin removed)
Salt and pepper as desired (sprinkle on the chicken)
1/2 cup chopped green onion
1/2 cup soy or tamari sauce
1/4 cup dry white wine
1/2 cup water
1/4 cup honey.

Put everything in a crockpot. Cook it for 3-4 hours on high. With one hour to go, make some high-in-fiber brown or wild rice. Put chicken pieces on top of rice and cover with sauce left in the crock pot.

Serves 8
427 calories, 8.1 grams of fat, 18% fat

•Do not overlook pre-packaged beans and rices that can be placed in a crock pot early in the morning and be ready for serving at night. I make a pot of beans every Sunday, use it throughout the week for a filling, virtually fat-free dish. If I have more than I need I share it with neighbors or freeze it for those occasions when I'm eating on the run.

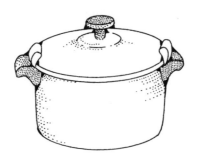

Despite the long list of ingredients, this turkey tetrazzini recipe is easy and fst to cook. It is a great way to use leftover turkey any time during the year. To save time start boiling the water for the spaghetti at the same time you begin sauteing the mushrooms. This dish freezes well and is an excellent candidate for doubling the recipe and freezing half for later use.

TURKEY TETRAZZINI

1/2 lb. sliced mushrooms
2 Tbs. flour
1/2 tsp. salt
1/2 tsp. ground black pepper
2 cups skim milk
1 tsp. Worcestershire
1/2 cup Lite Line or Weight Watcher's cheddar cheese
      product
1/2 cup scallions sliced
1 green pepper diced
2 pimentos finely chopped
1/2 lb. cooked spaghetti al dente, drained
2 cups cooked turkey cut into small cubes.
1/4 cup grated Parmesan cheese

In large non stick skillet or in your microwave, saute the mushrooms until tender. Stir in the flour, salt and pepper, then gradually add milk, stirring constantly to prevent lumps. Add Worcestershire sauce and simmer until somewhat thickened. Add cheese, green pepper, scallions and pimentos to sauce and mix well. Stir in turkey and spaghetti, combining mixture well. Pour into a 2 quart shallow casserole or baking dish that has been sprayed with a vegetable coating. Sprinkle the top of the casserole with Parmesan cheese. Bake casserole uncovered in preheated 350° oven about 20 minutes or until heated through.

195 calories, 5.5 grams of fat, 26% fat

CHICKEN AND SALSA VERDE CASSEROLE

2 medium diced onions
2 Tbs. chiccken stock
2 cups diced cooked chicken
1/2 cup Salsa Verde (store bought is fine)
8 oz. light cream cheese
12 6-inch corn tortillas
1 cup shredded reduced-calorie sharp cheddar sheese
1 cup part-skim milk mozzarella cheese

Saute onion in stock over medium heat until clear and beginning to brown, about 20 minutes. Remove pan from heat and add chicken, salsa and cream cheese. Mix lightly and season. Soften tortillas by wrapping in a damp cloth and then in foil, baking in a 350° oven for about 10 minutes or until done. Spray a 9" x 13" pan with vegetable coating. Alternate layers of tortillas, chicken mixture and cheese-finishing with tortillas and topping with cheese. Bake at 350° for 30 minutes.

8 servings
290 calories, 16 grams of fat, 50% fat

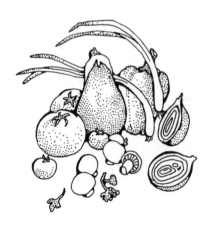

Where should I place this recipe? It uses chicken or fish or beef or pork. And, it is the most versatile recipe I can provide because you can put it together as many different ways as there are ingredients. I guess I'll just stick it in the middle.

MIX AND MATCH STIR FRY

1 16 oz. package of stir fry vegetables or purchase your own assortment*
1 pound boneless, skinless breast of chicken, sliced *or* lean flank steak, *or* sliced on diagonal *or lean* pork, sliced *or* scallops, shrimp *or* scampi *or* other fish suitable for stir fry
1 pkg frozen pea pods (optional)
2 tablespoons teriyaki or soy sauce or seasoning of your choice
2 tablespoons water
2-4 cups cooked brown rice, *or* pasta of your choice*

Heat frying pan, wok, or electric skillet on high. Spray surface with vegetable spray and add meat or fish and cook, stirring occasionally, until almost done. Remove from heat. Spray the skillet again and add the vegetables. Stir fry for about two minutes (time depends on amount of vegetables). Sprinkle teriyaki sauce and water over vegetables, reduce heat, and cover. Steam for 3-8 minutes (cook shorter for crisp vegetables, longer for softer vegetables). Return the meat, poultry or fish to the skillet. Put pea pods on top of mixture and steam for another two minutes. Serve over hot cooked rice or other pasta.
Serves 4-6 hearty eaters. Less than 20% fat

*any vegetable is suitable for stir fry. Cabbage, carrots, onions, water chestnuts, broccoli, and other vegetables that take longer to prepare can be cooked in the first stir fry/ steaming session and garlic, peppers and others that cook quickly added in the latter part of the cooking proces..

*try packaged, fresh or frozen whole wheat or spinach or other variety pastas to expand your choices.

BEEF TERIYAKI

1 lb. of low fat flank steak
3 cups mixed vegetables (broccoli, green beans, onions, red
  peppers)
1/3 cup teriyaki sauce.

Marinate flank steak in an oil-free Italian salad dressing.
Partially freeze beef to make it easy to cut on the bias into thin
strips.   Preheat teflon-lined wok or large skillet. Stir fry
frozen vegetables for 3-4 minutes or till crisp-tender. Remove vegetables from wok, but leave in any juices that may
have accumulated. Stir-cook the beef in the skillet until done.
Stir in teriyaki sauce and vegetables. Heat thoroughly.

Serve on rice (I use brown or wild rice because it's higher in
fiber).

4 servings
318 calories, 7.2 grams of fat, 21% fat

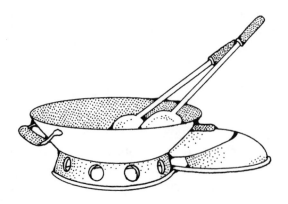

BEEF AND VEGETABLES

3/4 pound boneless beef top round steak
2 Tbs. teriyaki sauce
1 Tbs. water
2 tsp. sugar
1 1/2 tsp. cornstarch
Nonstick cooking spray
2 pkg. frozen pea pods
3 green onions sliced
1 tsp. minced garlic
1/4 lb. mushrooms, sliced
2 cups cooked brown rice

Partially freeze the beef then bias-slice it into thin strips. Combine the teriyaki sauce, water, sugar and cornstarch. Spray a skillet or wok with nonstick cooking spray. Preheat over high heat. Add the pea pods, mushrooms, onions and garlic. Cook and stir 2-3 minutes or until tender. Remove from skillet. Stir-fry the beef until tender then push it from the center of the skillet and add the teriyaki sauce. Cook and stir until the sauce until it's bubbly. Stir in the vegetable mixture and mix until it is heated through. Add cooked brown rice to the mixture. Serve.

Although it takes longer, you can also stir-fry the rice before adding the water and the rice will have a more crisp texture.

218 calories, 4.2 grams fat, 17% fat

The Worcestershire sauce contributes 260 mgm. of sodium to the recipe.

SHEPHERD'S PIE
Judy Wolson, Minneapolis

---

1 1/2 lbs. extra lean ground beef
1/2 cup tomato sauce
1 cup whole wheat bread crumbs
1 small onion chopped
1 egg white
1/8 tsp. pepper
1/2 tsp. salt
2 cups hot seasoned mashed potatoes (made with non fat
    milk)

Combine all ingredients except potatoes. Pack into a pie dish
and bake at 350° uncovered for 30 to 40 minutes or until done.
Cover with mashed potatoes, sprinkle the top with paprika
and place under broiler until potatoes brown–about 5 minutes.

8 servings
311 calories, 14.2 grams of fat, 42% fat

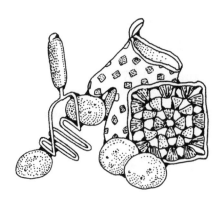

FISH HATERS FISH
Donna Lyman, Minneapolis

---

10 oz. turbot or sole
1 tsp. chicken bouillon
   (Pritikin non fat)
1 Tbs. minced dried onion
1 cucumber peeled and sliced
1 tomato, peeled and sliced.

Place fish in baking dish sprayed with Pam. Sprinkle with bouillon and onion and cover with slices of cucumber and tomato. Bake at 350° for 25 to 30 minutes.

2 servings
187 calories, 2.1 grams of fat, 12% fat

GRILLED SWORDFISH MARINATED IN LIME JUICE

3 lbs. swordfish steaks
2/3 cup lime juice
Olive oil

Marinate swordfish in lime juice in shallow glass bowl for several hours in the refrigerator, turning frequently. Brush steaks with olive oil and grill over hot coals., basting the steaks with marinade. The fish is cooked when it is firm to the touch and flakes easily with a fork. Serve with fresh tomato salsa.

6 servings
276 calories, 10 grams of fat, 34% fat

SEAFOOD CREOLE
Katherine Daline (Minneapolis)

1 Tbs. lite margarine (or butter)
1 cup sliced scallions
11/2 cup green pepper
2 cloves garlic, crushed
1 cup vegetable juice
2 med. tomatoes , blanched, peeled and chopped
2 Tbs. fresh parsley
2 tsp. paprika
1/2 tsp. sugar
1/8 tsp. red pepper
1 bay leaf, crumbled
1 1/2 Tbs. cornstarch, mixed with 1 Tbs. water
12 oz. peeled, deveined shrimp
12 oz. boneless cod, cut in 1" cubes.

In a non-stick coated pan, saute scallions, green pepper and crushed garlic until tender. Add the vegetable juice, tomatoes, parsley, paprika, sugar, red pepper and bay leaf. Cover and simmer for 30 minutes. Stir in the remaining ingredients. Bring to a boil. Reduce heat and simmer, stirring occasionally, until shrimp turn pink and mixture is thickened (about 7 minutes).

Serve over 2 cups of rice.

8 servings
187 calories, 3.4 grams of fat, 20% fat

CRAB STUFFED RED SNAPPER

2 lbs. red snapper
6 oz. cooked crabmeat or imitation crab meat, finely chopped
1/2 cup shredded carrot
1 thinly sliced green onion
1 tsp. sugar
1 tsp. cornstarch
1 tsp. soy sauce
1 tsp. dry sherry (optional)
1/4 cup dry sherry
1/4 cup soy sauce
1 Tbs. brown sugar
1 tsp. grated gingeroot
2 cups water

Score fish with diagonal cuts on each side, slicing almost through to the bone. Combine crabmeat, carrot, onion, sugar, cornstarch, 1 tsp. soy sauce and 1 tsp. sherry; spoon mixture into fish cavity, patting mixture to flatten evenly. Place fish on vegetable -sprayed rack of a poaching pan. Lower rack into pan or large kettle. Combine sherry, soy sauce, brown sugar, gingerroot, and 1 cup water. Pour over fish. Simmer, covered, twenty minutes or till fish flakes. Transfer fish to platter, spoon some liquid on top. Serves four.

Instead of red snapper you can also use perch or pike.

6 servings
211 calories, 2.7 grams of fat, 12% fat

The soy sauce makes it high in sodium.

If you have an appropriate serving dish, leave the head and tail on the fish for a more dramatic "presentation".

SALMON BAKED IN AN
ORANGE TARRAGON MARINADE

Allow 1/2–3/4 pound per person if using a whole salmon, because of bones, head, and tail.

Rub the filleted fish with orange juice concentrate and marinate over-night in the refrigerator.

To prepare fish for baking, preheat oven to 350°. Lay the fish on a cookie sheet that has been lined with foil. Rub additional marinade over and inside fish. Place thin slices of orange and sprigs of tarragon over and inside fish. To "steam" the fish while it bakes, cover it loosely with foil that has been folded to make a tent. Fish is done when firm to the touch or when it flakes easily or when a meat thermometer reaches 140–150°.

Serve the salmon with an orange sauce:

2 egg whites
1 cup non fat yogurt
1/4 cup tarragon vinegar
1/4 cup orange juice concentrate

In a blender or food processor fitted with a metal blade combine all ingredients and blend to the consistency of a sauce. Season with dill if desired.

This sauce recipe originally called for 1/2 cup of olive oil, added in a stream, during the mixing process. I think it works fine without the oil. Each teaspoon of oil adds 5 grams of fat to a recipe.

• 3 1/2 oz of broiled salmon has 7.4 grams of fat, 36% fat.
• 3 1/2 oz of raw chinook salmon has 14 grams of fat and is 60% fat.

LOWFAT SALMON RAMONOFF

6 oz. noodles, cooked*
1 cup plain yogurt, drained
1/2 package dry ranch-style dressing mix
10 oz. fresh salmon, cooked without fat**
1/2 cup fresh mushrooms
3 Tbs. chopped green onions
1/4 tsp. of dill weed

Combine all ingredients, mixing well. Put into a teflon coated or non-stick sprayed microwave-safe dish. Cook in microwave on medium-high until heated through (about five minutes). Stir and serve.

4 servings
233 calories, 6.3 grams of fat, 25% fat

*Use one of the many varieties of fresh pasta to make this dish special!

**You can also use drained of oil canned salmon or tuna.

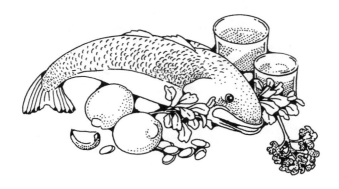

GRILLED SALMON FILLETS

1 lb. skinless boneless salmon fillets (about 1/2 inch thick)
2 Tbs. lemon juice
Fresh basil, crushed
1 Tbs. olive oil
1 Tbs. teriyaki sauce
1 tsp. Worcestershire sauce
1/2 tsp. minced garlic
1/4 tsp. pepper

Make sauce by combining lemon juice, basil, olive oil, teriyaki sauce, Worcestershire sauce, garlic and pepper in a small mixing bowl. Brush the sauce over the salmon. Grill over medium-hot coals for about five minutes or until salmon flakes easily when tested with a fork. Baste with sauce as it cooks.

4 servings
200 calories, 11 grams of fat, 50% fat

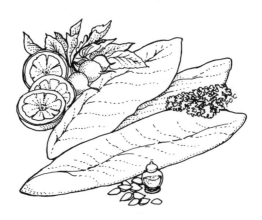

Don't be deceived by the ingredients or name of this dish. It is easy to fix and is delicious.

SHRIMP AND RICE

1 lb cleaned raw shrimp (about 2 cups)
2 Tbs. soy sauce
1 Tbs. sherry (optional)
1/2 tsp. ground ginger
1 1/2 cups sliced onion
1 cup celery sliced 1/4 inch diagonal
1 can sliced water chestnuts, drained
1 can bean sprouts, rinsed and drained
1 Tbs. cornstarch
1/2 tsp. dry non fat chicken broth mix
1/2 cup water
1 qt. cooked rice

In a large non-stick skillet combine and stir-cook shrimp, soy sauce, sherry and ginger over high heat until the shrimp are pink (about six minutes). Remove shrimp and set aside. In the same skillet, stir-cook onion, celery, water chestnuts and bean sprouts until the celery is crisp-tender (about six minutes). Mix the cornstarch, broth and water. Stir into the shrimp mixture. Cook, stirring constantly, until the mixture thickens and boils. Continue to cook one minute. Serve over rice.

8 servings
225 calories, 1 gram of fat, 4% fat

TUNAFISH CASSEROLE

2 cans water packed tuna, rinsed
1/2 cup 2% low fat cottage cheese
5 whole wheat bread slices, cubed

Sauce:
2 Tbs. margarine
3 Tbs. flour
1/2 cup low fat cheese (American flavor)
1 1/2 cup non-fat milk
1/2 tsp. salt
1 tsp. paprika

Mix tuna fish with cottage cheese and 1/2 of the cubed bread. Spread in 7' x 11' pan. Make sauce by melting margarine; add flour and stir. Add remaining ingredients and stir until heated and somewhat thick. Pour over tuna mixture. Toss remaining bread cubes with herb seasoning. Sprinkle over top. Bake at 350° for 25 minutes.

6 servings
95 calories, 3.72 grams of fat, 35% fat

Use 1% cottage cheese and Weight Watchers cheese to lower the fat to less than 20%.

Good for lunch or a light dinner.

Margaret Hancock is a Minneapolis area realtor who has less time for cooking than she would like, so the recipes I get from her are always easy and quick to fix. Pork products can be good choices for low fat eating because they are lower in fat than their reputation deserves. Cut even more time from the preparation by purchasing pre-trimmed and cut pork at your supermarket.

PORK / RICE / TOMATOES

6 pork chops or steaks trimmed of fat and cut into bite-size pieces.
2 cups brown rice, cooked.
Whole tomatoes, enough to balance.

Saute the pork bites for five minutes in non fat chicken broth. Mix with rice and tomatoes. Season with Italian seasonings to taste. Bake 1 hour at 350°.

250 calories, 10.5 grams of fat, 39% fat

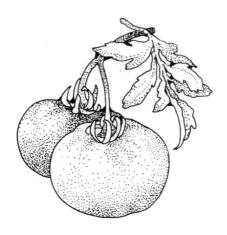

ZUCCHINI ITALIANO
Harriet Lesher, Portland

4 medium zucchini (about 1 1/2 lbs.)
1/2 lb. super lean ground beef (6% by weight)
1 clove garlic, minced
1 tsp. oregano
1 tsp. sweet basil
1 8 oz. can unsalted tomato sauce
3/4 cup low fat (1%) cottage cheese
2 egg whites
1/2 cup shredded part skim Mozzarella cheese, part skim

Cut zucchini in half lengthwise. Using a grapefruit spoon, scoop out interior of zucchini leaving a 1/4-inch shell. Turn shells cut side down in a 12" x 9" glass baking dish. Cover with wax paper. Microwave 5 minutes or until partially cooked. Let stand covered. Finely chop zucchini removed from centers. Crumble beef into a 1 quart measuring cup (or that size). Microwave 3 minutes or until meat is set, stirring once. Drain any fat. Stir in garlic, herbs, tomato sauce and chopped zucchini. Microwave, covered, 5 minutes. Combine cottage cheese and egg whites. Drain excess liquid from zucchini shells. Turn each shell cut side up in baking dish. Fill centers with cottage cheese mixture. Spoon meat mixture over zucchini. Cover with wax paper. Microwave 6–10 minutes or until heated through and zucchini shells are tender-crisp. Sprinkle with cheese. Microwave, uncovered, 2 minutes or until cheese is melted.

139 calories, 4 grams of fat, 26% fat

I was never very much of a fan of vegetarian chili until my friend, Helen Brown, brought this recipe by one day. There is no added fat so it's one of those recipes that is now a staple in my repertoire.

LOWFAT VEGETARIAN CHILI

32 oz. tomato juice
1 lg. can tomatoes
1 cup bulgar
1 onion
2 cloves garlic
3 carrots
1 tsp. cumin
1 tsp. basil
3 tsp. chili powder
dash Cayenne
2 cans kidney beans, drained
salt and pepper to taste

Boil tomato juice; add bulgar to it. Cover and cook until bulgar is not crunchy (about 15 minutes). Saute onion and garlic in a little water in a non-stick pan or in Lite olive oil. Add carrots and spices, cooking until tender. Add beans and other vegetables to tomato-bulgar mixture. Cook. Adjust spices. (I cheat with some packaged chili seasoning.)

6 servings
211 calories, 1.4 grams of fat, 5% fat

Just because this is here does not mean I believe it should be delegated to the last page of this section. I am betting that you will learn that sticking with something to the end will pay off. Read, check out your cupboards and try it.

MIX AND MATCH CANNED MEALS

These are the kinds of recipes that drive menu critics *CRAZY*. They are also the kinds of recipes that my lowfat lifestyle on the go fans *love*. Something happens when I open a couple of cans of somewhat non-descript foods and mix them together or add other touches that make them taste like a prepared from scratch meal. After you have tried these tap into your own intuitive mind and see what you can come up with.

NEW ENGLAND/PACIFIC NW CLAM CHOWDER

Instead of mixing a can of clam chowder with milk or cream: Empty a can of clam chowder soup into a large pot. Drain a can of chopped clams and measure the juice into the empty soup can. Fill to the top with condensed evaporated skim or two percent or skim milk. Add the milk/clam juice mixture to the soup. Heat slowly, stirring often. Add the clams. If the soup is too thick, add more milk. Serve with crusty whole wheat bread and a tossed green salad.

AND/OR
Mix low fat chili with vegetable or minestrone soup.
Mix homemade macaroni and cheese with frozen peas with pearl onions and water packed tuna.
Mix one can Stagg Chicken or Beef Chili and one can (any variety) of Progresso soup.
Add a can of mixed vegetables to canned tomato soup.

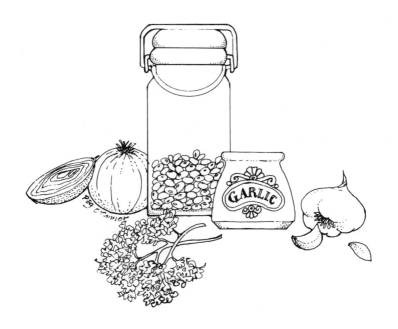

ON THE SIDE
(Vegetable, Rice and Pasta Recipes)

I am a proponent of serving vegetable dishes mixed with small portions of meat as opposed to meat with vegetable dishes "on the side". With some ingenuity and a mental framework that says, "make changes slowly." even die-hard meat and potatoes families have discovered their diets can evolve to be more in keeping with U. S. Dietary Goals that encourage more of these fiber-filled side dishes. We now know that it is not carbohydrates that are the culprits in high fat eating. It is the fat in the sauces we put on the pastas, rice and other vegetable dishes. Here are some of my favorite side dishes.

ORANGE PINEAPPLE SWEET POTATOES
Judy Wolson (Minneapolis)

12 oz. peeled hot cooked sweet potatoes
2 cups hot cooked sliced carrots
1 cup canned crushed pineapple (no sugar added)
2 Tbs. plus 2 tsp. reduced calorie orange marmalade
1 tsp. grated orange rind
1/4 tsp ground cinnamon
Dash of salt.

Mash potatoes and carrots together. Add remaining ingredients. Stir to combine, put into a casserole and bake at 375° for 30 minutes.

6 servings
100 calories, 1 gram of fat, 9% fat.

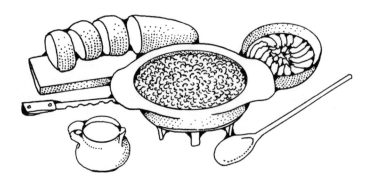

LATKES (Potato Pancakes)
Jackie Harris (Minneapolis)

---

3 large potatoes, peeled and grated*
1/4 cup grated onion
2 egg whites
1/2 tsp. salt
1/4 tsp. baking powder (optional)
3 Tbs. matzo meal or all purpose flour

Put the potatoes in a mixing bowl and add the onion and beaten egg white. Mix well. Combine salt, baking powder, matzo meal or flour, and slowly add to potato mixture. Mix thoroughly. Drop the mixture by tablespoonfuls onto a heated skillet that's been sprayed with vegetable coating. Cook on one side until well browned, turn over and brown on second side. Serve with unsweetened applesauce.

*Grate the potatoes in a food processor and then add the other ingredients.

Makes 16 pancakes.

Each serving is 70 calories, less than 1 gm fat, 1% fat.

• Cover potatoes with water to keep them from turning black while you are fixing them.

> *"Beans, beans, the body's musical fruit—*
> *the more you eat, the more you toot!*
> *The more you toot, the better you feel,*
> *so why not eat beans at every meal?"*

I hope you are not offended, but there is no way to get around it. Beans make us gassy. We are one of the few cultures where it is "not cool" to get rid of intestinal gas. I always tell my audiences that we have to quit "fighting the fart" and remember the adage, "life is a gas!"

Some beans will affect some people in some ways and others in other ways. For example, I can eat kidney beans, green beans, garbanzos and limas with no trouble, but give me black or navy beans and it's rocket time. You have probably done your own research on beans and your body. There are so many varieties I know you can find a few that are suitable for your personal taste.

• DE-GASSING BEANS

To decrease the flatulence (gas) that usually accompanies eating beans, soak the beans overnight–throw out the water (sugars that would ferment in the intestines) and soak again. The more often you do this, the less gassy the beans will be. You can also boil beans for one minute and let them sit in the water for sixty minutes to hasten the de-gassing process.

• Other hints that are for the beans...
Lentils, limas and split peas produce less flatulence.
Garbanzos take the longest to cook.
For some reason, canned beans usually don't cause as much intestinal gas as beans "from scratch".
Many recipes call for adding fat to beans to decrease the foaming that often accompanies cooking beans. Remember that this adds fat. You are better off to skim the foam as the beans cook.
Add acidic foods that take a long time to cook (i. e. tomatoes, onions) after you cook beans.

SPICY BLACK BEANS

2 garlic cloves, chopped
1 lb. black beans
Water
2 cups chicken stock
Salt and pepper
2 Tbs. dry vermouth
1 tsp. cumin
Tabasco
Optional: cornstarch

Soak beans overnight or, for a quicker method, cover beans with water, bring to boil for 1 minute, then let sit in covered pot for 1 hour. Drain. Combine the beans, 6 cups fresh water, stock, garlic, and a pinch of salt in a large saucepan and bring to a boil. Reduce heat, and simmer, partially covered, until tender, about 1 1/2 hours. Stir in remaining ingredients.

Serves 8
126 calories, .6 grams of fat, 4% fat

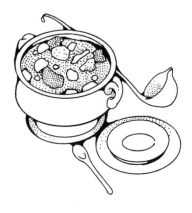

LENTIL AND RICE CASSEROLE

2/3 cup dried lentils
1 cup rice
1 onion, diced
1 clove garlic, minced
5 stalks celery, diced
1 28-oz. can crushed tomatoes in sauce
1 tsp. dried thyme
1/2 tsp. salt
1/4 tsp. white pepper
1 tsp. dried dill weed
1/2 cup bread crumbs

Soak lentils in water overnight. Pour out the water and replace it with fresh water to cover. Simmer slowly until lentils are tender, about 2 hours. Place rice and 3 cups water in a saucepan, bring to a boil, then cover and simmer for 20 minutes. While the rice cooks, saute onion, garlic and celery in 1/4 cup water or non-fat bouillon until soft. Add tomatoes, drained lentils, 1/2 cup lentil cooking water, rice, and spices. Mix well and pour into a 2-quart non-stick baking pan. Sprinkle with bread crumbs and bake at 350° for 30 minutes.

6 servings
217 calories, 1 gram fat, 3% fat

VEGETARIAN LENTIL DISH
Helene Horton (Hawaii)

1 onion, chopped
2 cloves of garlic, minced
5-6 large sliced mushrooms
1/4 cup pearl barley
1 tsp. cumin
juice from 1/2 lemon.
Salt and pepper to taste
3/4 cup lentils
2 cups water

Saute the chopped onions in chicken broth or water. Add garlic and mushrooms and stir. Add pearl barley, cumin and stir with lemon juice and salt and pepper to taste. Add 2 cups of water and the lentils. Cover and cook slowly for one hour (Check it regularly, as you may need to add more water).

2 servings
154 calories , .8 grams of fat, 2% fat

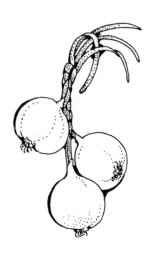

VEGETABLE LASAGNE

This is a lasagne that with a little innovation and a lot of leftover vegetables can be made no two ways twice!

3 cups tomato paste
1 Tbs. basil
1 Tbs. oregano
2 tsp. chopped garlic
1/2 cup water
Salt and pepper
1 eggplant
1 lb. zucchini, sliced thinly
1/2 lb. mushrooms, sliced
1/2 Tbs. basil
Scant olive oil
1 pint low fat cottage cheese
2 cups skim-milk mozzarella
1 cup grated Parmesan cheese
1 lb. fresh or canned Italian tomatoes, sliced

Preheat oven to 350°. Combine tomato paste, basil, oregano, garlic, water, salt and pepper in a sauce pan and simmer over low heat for 20–25 minutes, stirring often to prevent burning. Soften eggplant in a saute pan with 1/2 cup of water or stock. Heat olive oil in the saute pan and saute zucchini, mushrooms, and basil until vegetables are softened.

To assemble the lasagna, spread a small amount of tomato sauce in a 9 x 11 dish. Place a layer of noodles on top of the sauce and spread with tomato sauce. Put eggplant slices on the sauce and then a third of the cottage cheese, mozzarella and Parmesan. Repeat the layering process with the zucchini-mushroom mixture and finish the last layer with the cheeses. Bake covered with non-stick sprayed foil for 1 hour. Remove foil and bake at 400° for 15–20 minutes.

8 servings
247 calories, 10 grams of fat, 27% fat

RISI E BISI (Italian rice and peas)

1/2 cup hot, firm-cooked brown rice
1/4 cup boiling water
1 envelope instant chicken broth and seasoning mix
1/2 tsp. dehydrated onion flakes
1 tsp. minced parsley
Pepper
Few drops of sherry extract
4 oz. uncooked peas.

Combine all ingredients in a small saucepan. Bring to a boil,
reduce heat, cover and simmer 15 minutes or until the peas
are soft. If the peas and rice are too moist, remove the cover
and continue cooking.

One serving!
238 calories, 2 grams fat, 9% fat

SPANISH RICE (made using the above dish)

In a saucepan combine:
Risi and Bisi (above)
 3/4 cup tomato juice

1/2 tsp. Worcestershire sauce
1/2 diced medium green pepper
1/2 shredded pimento
1/2 cup diced celery
Dash of Cayenne pepper.

Cook until vegetables are sauce. Add Risi and heat.

2 servings
272 calories, 5 grams fat, 8% fat

This is a Southern specialty.

HOPPIN JOHN

2 cups cooked rice
1 1/4 cups black-eyed peas
Water
2 cloves of garlic, chopped
1 bay leaf
salt and pepper
Chopped green and red bell peppers
Chopped red onion

Place peas in a large saucepan and add just enough water to cover. With a lid on the pan, bring to a boil and let boil for 1 minute. Remove from heat and let stand for one hour. Drain, then add fresh water–enough to cover peas with an inch of water. (At this stage you may add chicken or vegetable stock, which will give the peas more flavor). Add onion, garlic, bay leaf, salt and pepper. Bring to a boil and then cover and simmer for 1–2 hours or until you can slightly mash peas with a fork. Add rice to peas and serve with chopped bell peppers and onion.

8 servings
70 calories, less than 1 gram of fat, 2% fat

This dish takes a little more time to prepare, but is well worth it. With a salad and some fresh hot bread this "side dish" makes a complete low fat, high fiber meal.

ZINGY STUFFED ZUCCHINI
Bev Holtzer (Kansas City)

---

6 medium zucchini (about 1 1/2 pounds)
1 clove of garlic, split
Scant margarine
1 medium onion, chopped
1 cup fresh tomatoes, chopped
1 cup cooked brown rice
1/2 tsp. dried oregano
1 tsp. salt
1/4 tsp. cayenne (optional)
1/2 cup grated Parmesan

Preheat oven to 450°. Wash zucchini; cut off stems, cut each in half lengthwise. In a small amount of boiling water, cook the zucchini, covered, for five minutes or until tender. Drain well, cool, scoop out the seeds. In a scant amount of margarine or oil saute garlic until golden; lift out and discard the garlic (save the drippings). Add onion, saute, stirring until golden. Add tomato, rice, oregano and cayenne. Toss with a fork to mix well. Sprinkle the inside of each zucchini with salt and pepper and add the rice mixture. Sprinkle the top with Parmesan cheese. Arrange in a single layer in a baking dish. Bake uncovered for 15 minutes. Place under the broiler several minutes to brown the top. <u>Be careful not to burn!</u>

6 servings
105 calories, 5 grams fat, 34% fat

This makes a great low-cal, fat-free side dish, hot or cold.

RATATOUILLE

In a Dutch oven, combine your vegetable favorites   diced into small pieces. Add a large can of tomato juice and simmer until done:

Suggested vegetables: eggplant (with skin), zucchini, celery, onion, green pepper, cabbage, carrots, mushrooms, and diced fresh or canned tomatoes.

Be generous with seasonings, especially oregano, garlic powder, and pepper. Use other seasonings as desired.

Serving size depends on vegetables used.
Each 1/2 cup serving is 30 calories and less than 1 gm. of fat.

MEXICAN EGGPLANT

1 medium eggplant, peeled and cut into cubes
1 can (15 oz) of tomatoes or
4 medium fresh tomatoes, peeled and chopped
1 clove of garlic, minced
2 Tbsp. chopped onion
1/4 tsp. chili powder
Dash of pepper

Combine all ingredients in a skillet and simmer gently 15-20 minutes or until the eggplant is tender.

4 servings
Each serving is 55 calories and has less than 1 gm. fat.

GRILLED VEGETABLES WITH BASIL SAUCE

For the Basil Sauce:
2 egg whites
5 tsp. lemon juice
1 tsp. Dijon mustard
3/4 fresh basil leaves
1/4 tsp. salt
1/4 tsp. white pepper
2 T. olive oil

Make the basil sauce in a food processor. With the motor running, blend the egg, lemon juice, mustard, basil, salt and pepper. Add the oil, blending the mixture until it is thickened. Can be made a day in advance.

6 green onions, cut in 1-inch pieces
8 cherry tomatoes
1 red bell pepper, quartered
1 green or yellow bell pepper, quartered
1 zucchini, cut in 1/4-inch rounds
1 yellow squash, cut in 1/4-inch rounds
8 mushrooms

Skewer the vegetables on wooden skewers that have been soaked in water for 20 minutes. Brush the vegetables with olive oil so they do not stick to grill. Grill over glowing coals, turning once.

6 servings

102 calories,2,6 grams fat, 22% fat
(All the fat comes from the olive oil .)

HEAVENLY PASTA

4 oz. angel hair pasta, cooked
two Weight Watchers cheese slices
2 Tbs. skim milk or yogurt

Melt cheese on pasta in microwave and add the yogurt or milk to cool it. Sprinkle with dill/onion seasoning and Molly Sour Cream Mcbutter.

1 serving
114 calories, 4 grams fat, 32 % fat

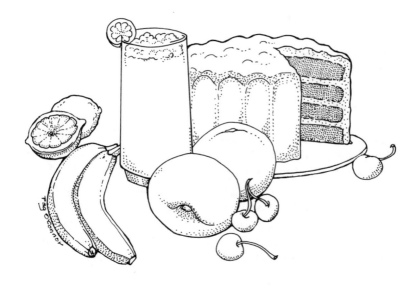

SWEET TREATS

If you have a sweet tooth you may have searched out this section first. It is short (but sweet) and includes recipes that have pleased the palate of my family and friends. I have also included sweet beverages that satisfy me between meals and are also teriffic for a meal on the run.

Non fat frozen yogurt and fresh fruit and low fat cookies are the wisest choices for lowfat desserts. BUT, when I eat out at a restaurant that specializes in desserts I take advantage of their chef's expertise and enjoy myself. In fact my friends and I usually create a dessert feast by ordering a variety from the menu and sharing them with one another. It is a whole new way to party.

I have also included sweet beverages that satisfy me between meals and work great for non-fat energy on the go.

LOWFAT ICE CREAM BALLS

1 quart frozen non fat yogurt
1 package Jello Sugar Free Chocolate Pudding
1 cup evaporated skim milk
1 cup water

Allow frozen non fat yogurt to soften slightly. Mix the chocolate pudding with the evaporated skim milk and water. Beat the mixture well. Using two spoons, form balls of the frozen yogurt. (They won't be perfect). Put them on a platter. Lightly ice the balls with the chocolate pudding and put them in the freezer. (If you put too much pudding on the ice cream balls, they're too hard to eat later!) Make only six at a time so they don't melt. When frozen solid, serve.

8 one-half cup servings
Each serving is 67 calories and has negligible fat.

FROZEN DESSERT CAKE

One angel food cake
One pint of non fat frozen yogurt, vanilla or the flavor of your choice.
Jello Sugar Free Chocolate Pudding.

Cut the cake horizontally in two. Spread 1 inch of softened non fat frozen yogurt between the layers. Ice cake with the chocolate pudding. Freeze.

12 serving
Each serving is 215 calories and has negligible fat.

LOWFAT BAKED ALASKA

For an elegant presentation, serve this on a glass cake plate but be sure it is one you can put in a hot oven for one minute (when you brown the meringue).

1 pint chocolate non fat frozen yogurt, slightly softened
1 pint strawberry non fat frozen yogurt or sorbet, slightly softened
Angel food cake cut in two layers
5 egg whites
1/2 tsp. cream of tartar
1 tsp. vanilla extract
1/4 cup of sugar

Use two 8-inch Teflon coated cake pans or line two regular cake pans with wax paper, leaving an overhang around the edges. Spread the chocolate nonfat yogurt evenly into one pan and the strawberry into the other. Freeze until each is firm. Place one layer of the cake on your serving dish. Invert the chocolate yogurt on the cake then repeat with the strawberry layer. Cover with second layer of cake. Beat room temperature egg whites until foamy. Add cream of tartar and vanilla, and beat until soft peaks form. Gradually add sugar, one tablespoon at a time, beat until stiff peaks form. Remove layers from freezer and quickly spread meringue over entire surface, making sure edges are sealed to the serving plate. Bake at 475o for one minute or until meringue peaks are lightly browned. Slice into wedges, and serve immediately.

12 servings.
Each serving is 180 calories and has negligible fat.

NUCLEAR CAKE

I often lecture about "nuking" cakes. That means I put ingredients in a microwave, step back and hope for the best. There have been some incredible successes with this method and there have also been some DISASTERS. Jeannie Morris gave me the following recipe for a cake which I modified and put in my microwave for a quick-to-fix dessert or snack. (My classes don't believe this works and refuse to try it until they see it demonstrated and served in my home!)

Mix 1 package of Jiffy corn muffin mix with
1 package of yellow cake mix and
3-5 egg whites and
sparkling water or diet 7-up to moisten to cake cooking consistency.

Place the ingredients in a glass bowl or dish that's been sprayed with vegetable spray. Bake in your oven or microwave until it has the consistency of cake! While hot, cover with non fat frozen yogurt (any flavor), pudding or cool slightly and serve with fresh fruit.

(These is one of those recipes that drive gourmet cooks crazy.)

• Use vanilla flavored yogurt to make yogurt cheese. (See page 27.) Mix it with low fat whipped cream cheese as a sauce for fruit salads and as topping for non fat yogurts and cakes.

• Apple and pear slices are the most satisfying snack you can carry in a car cooler. You will never have to miss a meal. Preparation can be a breeze if you have a fruit wedger. This easy-to-store utensil cores and wedges these fruits into even slices in one swift motion.

BEV'S LOWER IN FAT CHEESECAKE
Bev Holtzer, Kansas City

---

4 cups skim milk ricotta cheese
5 egg whites, 2 egg yolks
1 cup non fat buttermilk
1/2 cup (or less) of sugar
1 Tbs. cornstarch
2 tsps. vanilla extract
1/4 tsp. salt
juice and grated rind of one small lemon

In a large bowl beat ricotta cheese until smooth. Add egg yolks one at a time, beating well after each addition. Add buttermilk, sugar, cornstarch, vanilla, salt and lemon juice and rind. Slowly pour in egg whites and beat until the mixture is thick. Pour the batter into a springform pan that has been sprayed with vegetable spray. Bake in a preheated 375 degree oven for one hour. Cool completely before serving. If desired, garnish with fresh fruit or fruit flavored yogurt or frost with flavored yogurt cheese.

12 servings
Each is 172 calories, 7.6 g. fat, 39% fat

•To release more juice from lemons, before cutting and squeezing, let them come to room temperature or microwave them for one minute on medium power.

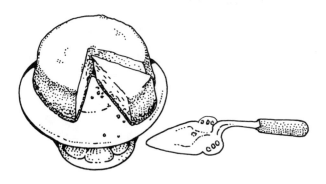

ANOTHER CHEESECAKE

1 1/4 cup graham cracker crumbs
1/4 cup melted margarine.
8 oz. light cream cheese
1/2 cup sugar
5 egg whites
1 pint nonfat vanilla yogurt cheese (page 27)
1 tsp. vanilla

Mix crumbs and margarine. Press to bottom and sides of 9"
pie plate that has been sprayed with vegetable coating. Mix
cream cheese, sugar, and egg whites together until smooth
using blender or food processor. Pour into pie crust. Bake at
350o for 20 minutes. Cool. Mix yogurt cheese and vanilla
together. Pour over cooked cream cheese mixture. Bake at
350o for another 20 minutes. Chill well before serving.

Makes 12 servings
133 calories, 7.2 grams of fat, 47% fat
(Regular cheesecake is 257 calories 16.3 grams of fat 58% fat.)

•Use vanilla flavored yogurt to make yogurt cheese (Page
27). Mix it with light cream cheese and use it to top graham
crackers, fresh or froxen fruit or non fat frozen yogurt..

•Have old bananas on hand? Freeze them and mix them in
the blender with the flavored yogurt of your choice. Add a
dash of vanilla. You will have a delicious dessert.

ICE DESSERTS

STRAWBERRY ICE
3 pints strawberries
2 bananas
2 Tbs. sugar

PINEAPPLE ICE
1 pineapple
juice of one lemon
2 Tbs. sugar

KIWI ICE
12 kiwi
juice of one lime
juice of one lemon
2 Tbs. of sugar

MELON ICE
4 cups watermelon (seeds removed)
2 Tbs. sugar
2 Tbs. lemon juice

You will need a food processor for these fat free icy desserts. Blend the fruits in a food processor until thoroughly pureed. Add the lemon and sugar to prevent discoloration. Remove from processor to tray for freezing. When almost frozen return to food processor and puree again. Repeat the puree/freeze process at least one more time (this prevents crystals from forming in the ice). Serve and enjoy!

Each 1/2 cup serving is 60 calories or less and has negligible fat.

CANTALOPE SLUSH

1/2 cantalope
1 cup skim milk
1 cup orange non fat frozen yogurt

Prepare ahead: Cut 1/2 cantalope into small round balls. Freeze.
In a blender, combine frozen melon balls, 1 cup skim milk and blend. Add non fat yogurt a spoonful at a time, blending until slushy.

4 servings
Each serving is 75 calories and has negligible fat.

RONDA'S SMOOTHIE

4 fresh peaches (or 1 pint strawberries)
2 ripe bananas
1 8 oz. carton vanilla non-fat yogurt
1 cup non fat milk

Cut fresh fruit into small pieces and put into a blender. Blend. Add the non-fat yogurt and milk and blend again. You can make the drink more icy by blending the fruit with chopped ice.

8 servings
Each serving is 70 calories and has negligible fat.

Is there such a thing as low fat egg nog? Barb Garrett from Minnesota brought this to me at holiday time. It's not the real thing, but an excellent substitute–especially when you consider it is non-fat. The class decided that a reasonable alternative might be mixing "the real thing" half and half with this mixture. Turned out to be a great idea. I have added it to desserts because it is so sweet.

EGG NOG

Blend at high speed in blender until smooth:

1 1/2 cups skim milk
1 1/2 tsp. vanilla extract
1/3 cup nonfat dry milk
1/2 tsp nutmeg
2 Tbs. sugar
1/8 tsp salt
4 ice cubes

This makes 4 cups.
Each serving is 80 calories, 0 fat compared to 240 calories per cup, 6 grams of fat in "the real thing."

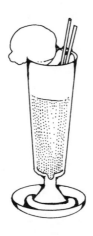

OTHER RECOMMENDED COOKBOOKS

I am often asked to recommend a cookbook that goes beyond the recipes you found here. When I first started cooking the low fat way the selection was limited. That has changed. Major and minor publishing house and people like myself have spent hours modifying old recipes and developing new ones. The following list includes the cookbooks that are my favorites. If you cannot find them in your local store, write to me c/o Lifestyles by Ronda Gates, P. O. Box 1843, Lake Oswego, OR 97035, for purchasing information.

The Lowfat Lifestyle by Ronda Gates and Valerie Parker
Living Lean and Loving It by Eve Lowry, R. D. and Carla
       Mulligan-Ennis
Microwaving Light and Healthy by Barbara Methven
Cooking Light by Susan McIntosh
Spa Specialties by Deborah Hart
Don't Eat Your Heart Out by Joseph C. Piscatella
Weight Watchers Quick Start Plus Program Cookbook
Weight Watchers Quick and Easy Menu Book
Jane Brody's Good Food Book by Jane Brody
New American Diet by Sonja Connor, R. D. and William E.
       Connor, M. D.
Low-Fat, Low-Cholesterol Cookbook by American Heart
       Association

OTHER VALUABLE REFERENCES
The Food Book
The Fast Food Guide by Jacobsen and Fritschner
Food Values of Portions Commonly Used by Pennington and
       Church

STOP!

I'll bet you thought you were only half way through the book. You may have turned the page wondering what you would read about next.

You *are* half way through the book and you *are* finished with Changes and Bites. And, you are *not* finished. If you turn the page, you will discover the rest of the book is upside down. How could the publisher have made such a serious error?

There are no mistakes. Everything happens for a reason.

Changes occur when people are uncomfortable with their life. Their discomforture generates emotions. Author John Bradshaw breaks the word emotions down so the E stands for energy–energy in motion generates change. In time, in addition to their well being they become more interested in being well. They want to understand how to apply the principles of living that assure optimum health. They take bites of new recipes. Soon they also want to know about Nutrition–and More.

So, turn the book over and begin again. You will find (Nuggets of) Nutrition and More about these learnings.

TO ORDER ADDITIONAL COPIES OF

Nutrition Nuggets And More by Ronda Gates
or
The Lowfat Lifestyle by Ronda Gates and Valerie Parker
or
Lifestyles Resource Guide by Ronda Gates

Send check or money order to:
 Lifestyles 4 Heart Press
 P. O. Box 1843
 Lake Oswego, OR 97035

--------------------------------**clip here**-----------------------------
NAME_____
ADDRESS_____
CITY_____STATE_____ZIP_____

Quantity:
_____Nutrition Nuggets And More $10.95
_____The Lowfat Lifestyle (paperback) $ 9.95
_____The Lowfat Lifestyle (spiral bound) $11.95
_____Lifestyles Resource Guide $ 5.00
Add $1.50 per book for shipping and handling
AMOUNT ENCLOSED:_____

--------------------------------**clip here**-----------------------------
NAME_____
ADDRESS_____
CITY_____STATE_____ZIP_____

Quantity:
_____Nutrition Nuggets And More $10.95
_____The Lowfat Lifestyle (paperback) $ 9.95
_____The Lowfat Lifestyle (spiral bound) $11.95
_____Lifestyles Resource Guide $ 5.00
Add $1.50 per book for shipping and handling
AMOUNT ENCLOSED:_____

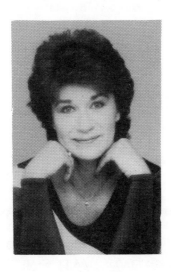

ABOUT RONDA GATES

Ronda Gates, M. S. is president of LIFESTYLES by Ronda Gates, a corporation that provides a variety of health promotion lectures, workshops, courses, seminars and products to the public, corporate, educational and industrial community. She is best known as an entertaining speaker who brings common sense to the often confusing and quickly evolving information about exercise, nutrition, weight management and behaviors associated with lifestyle change.

Ronda has produced two slide shows and videos, Label Fables and Lowfat Lifestyle® on the Go, and is co-author with Valerie Parker of The Lowfat Lifestyle®, which has sold more than 35,000 copies. While associated with nutritional biochemist Covert Bailey, M. S., Ronda was instrumental in the development of his Fit Or Fat® System.

For additional information about Ronda and/or the products and services she and her company provide write LIFESTYLES by Ronda Gates, P. O. Box 1843, Lake Oswego, OR 97035 or call 503-620-3233